The Psychobiology of Transsexualism and Transgenderism

The Psychobiology of Transsexualism and Transgenderism

A New View Based on Scientific Evidence

Thomas E. Bevan, PhD

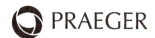

PRAEGER

AN IMPRINT OF ABC-CLIO, LLC
Santa Barbara, California • Denver, Colorado • Oxford, England

Library of Congress Cataloging-in-Publication Data

Bevan, Thomas E., author.
 The psychobiology of transsexualism and transgenderism : a new view based on scientific evidence / Thomas E. Bevan.
   p.; cm.
 Includes bibliographical references and index.
 ISBN 978-1-4408-3126-3 (alk. paper) – ISBN 978-1-4408-3127-0 (ebook)
 I. Title.
 [DNLM: 1. Transsexualism–etiology. 2. Sexuality–psychology. 3. Transgendered Persons–psychology. 4. Transsexualism–genetics. 5. Transsexualism–physiopathology. WM 611]
   RC560.G45   2015
   616.6′900867–dc23   2014024279

ISBN: 978-1-4408-3126-3
EISBN: 978-1-4408-3127-0

19 18 17 16 15   1 2 3 4 5

This book is also available on the World Wide Web as an eBook.
Visit www.abc-clio.com for details.

Praeger
An Imprint of ABC-CLIO, LLC

ABC-CLIO, LLC
130 Cremona Drive, P.O. Box 1911
Santa Barbara, California 93116-1911

This book is printed on acid-free paper ∞
Manufactured in the United States of America

This book discusses treatments (including types of medication and mental health therapies), diagnostic tests for various symptoms and mental health problems, and organizations. The author has made every effort to present accurate and up-to-date information. However, the information in this book is not intended to recommend or endorse particular treatments or organizations, or substitute for the care or medical advice of a qualified health professional, or used to alter any medical therapy without a medical doctor's advice. Specific situations may require specific therapeutic approaches not included in this book. For those reasons, we recommend that readers follow the advice of qualified health care professionals directly involved in their care. Readers who suspect they may have specific medical problems should consult a physician about any suggestions made in this book.

I dedicate this book to my mentor, Julian Jaynes, to my children, and to the love of my life, my darling wife.

Contents

Tables and Figures

Tables

Figures

Preface

We struggle against it, we fight to deny it, but it is of course pretense, it is a lie. Beneath our poised appearance, the truth is we are completely out of control. Causality. There is no escape from it, we are forever slaves to it. Our only hope, our only peace is to understand it, to understand the "why." "Why" is what separates us from them, you from me. "Why" is the only real power, without it you are powerless.

—*The Merovingian in* The Matrix Reloaded

There are lots of "whys" about transsexualism and transgenderism.

Why should a seemingly normal person risk their career, reputation, and family by cross-dressing in secret? Why do some people permanently change their bodies to be more like another sex and thus to better assume a different gender? Why do both types of people risk bullying, physical danger, abuse, and rejection? Why do they tolerate the long-term effects of having a secret life that produce preoccupation, inauthenticity, and depression? These "whys" are only the top-level of a hierarchy of whys.

As the quote that opens this preface indicates, we are all out of control at the subconscious level. We have no conscious sensation and control of many of the functions of our brains and nervous systems. If we did, we would probably need a brain many times its current size to accommodate all that processing. We would be overwhelmed in thought by our own internal processes. The quote of course is from a movie written in part by Larry, now Lana, Wachowski as influenced by the Kevin Kelly book *Out of Control*. Kevin Kelly is the founding editor of *Wired* Magazine and was interested in the similarity between biological systems and computer network systems, both having subordinate widgets and functions that the whole system cannot control.

So the overall question is why do transsexuals and transgender people do what they do despite wholesale cultural rejection? As detailed in this book, these behaviors have a biological basis. The evidence for this biological basis is currently spread across some 22 scientific disciplines. Everyone has at least one biological gender predisposition. Gender behavior categories are constructed by culture and vary from culture to culture in terms of number, behaviors, and flexibility. A person's gender behavior disposition may be incongruent with a person's culturally assigned gender behavior category. This incongruency results in transsexual and transgender behavior in which a person acts in a different gender behavior category from that assigned. In most binary gender system cultures, there are only two gender behavior categories, man and woman, but in some cultures there are four or five categories.

Gender predisposition is a widget or a mechanism that we cannot control. It always gets a vote on our behavior starting at 3 to 4 years old when realization of transsexual and transgender behavior begins.

Understanding the biological basis and the biopsychology of transsexualism and transgenderism (TSTG) provides us with power. Without this understanding, we lack the stronger power to appropriately set or change governmental, medical, and cultural policies and attitudes regarding TSTG. Without this understanding, we do not have the power to fully understand the human condition.

Acknowledgments

I acknowledge the assistance and understanding of V. E., Genny Jacks, and Patricia Bell.

Definitions and Acronyms

AIS	Androgen insensitivity syndrome
Amygdala	Brain structure controlling emotion
AR	Androgen receptor gene
Aromatase	Enzyme that catalyzes testosterone into dihydrotestosterone
Autism spectrum	Group of neurodevelopmental phenomena
Autogynephilia	Love of oneself as a woman
Bakla	Gender behavior category in Philippines
Binary gender system	System with two gender behavior categories
BNST	Bed nucleus of the stria terminalis
Boy/man	Masculine gender terms in binary gender system
Bugis	Indonesian subculture with five gender behavior categories
CAH	Congenital adrenal hyperplasia
Castrati	Boys castrated in childhood to preserve a soprano/contralto singing voice
Cisgender	Gender category in alignment with sex
Consanguinity	Having children with a close relative
Corpus callosum	Major structure connecting brain hemispheres
Cross-dresser	One who dresses in clothes of nonassigned gender behavior category

Cross-dressing	Dressing in clothes of nonassigned gender behavior category
DES	Diethylstilbestrol, a drug formerly given to prevent miscarriages suspected of causing TSTG
Dizygotic twins	Nonidentical in terms of DNA at conception
Drag	Cross-dressing for performance
DSD	Differences in sexual development, intersex
DSM-V	*Diagnostic and Statistical Manual,* 5th edition
DTI-MRI	Diffusion tensor imaging magnetic resonance imaging
EEG	Electroencephalogram, transduction of minute electrical signals from the scalp reflecting brain activity
Existential crisis	Life change that tends to change behavior
Fa'afafine	Samoan gender behavior category
Feminization surgery	Surgery to increase female appearance
fMRI	Functional magnetic resonance imaging
FTM	Female-to-male transsexual and transgender
Gender	Behaviors within gender behavior category
Gender behavior category	Set of behaviors determined by culture
Gender behavior predisposition	Biological predisposition with regard to gender behavior categories
Gender confirmation surgery	Misnomer for TS GPS
Gender constancy	Ability to infer sex from gender presentation
Gender dysphoria	Unhappiness with assigned gender behavior category
Gender identity	Verbalization of congruent gender behavior category
Gender identity disorder (GID)	Pathological term for TSTG
Genderqueer	Those not having a congruent gender behavior category
Gender reconstruction surgery	Misnomer for TS GPS

Gender system	System of gender behavior categories
Girl/woman	Feminine gender terms in binary gender system
GLBT	Gay, lesbian, bisexual, and transgender
GnRH	Gonadotropin-releasing hormone
Gray matter	Brain matter primarily containing neuron and other cell bodies
Handedness	Preference for use of left or right hand for particular tasks
HBIGDA	Former name of WPATH
Hijra	TSTG subculture in South Asia
HRT	Hormone-replacement therapy; old name for hormone therapy
HT	Hormone therapy
ICD-10	*International Classification of Diseases,* Version 10
INAH	Interstitial nucleus of anterior hypothalamus
Intersex	Difference in sexual development
Kallmann syndrome	Genetic defect resulting in low testosterone levels
Kathoey	MTF TSTG from Thailand
Lhamana	Zuni gender behavior category
Mahu	Hawaiian gender behavior category
Masculinization surgery	Surgery to increase male appearance
Monozygotic twins	Twins having identical DNA at conception
Mosaicism	Having more than one DNA species
MRI	Magnetic Resonance Imaging
MTF	Male-to-female transsexual or transgender
Muxe	Mexican gender behavior category
Nadleehi	Navajo gender behavior category
Nonbinary gender system	Gender system having other than two gender behavior categories
Operationalization	Reducing theory to testable experimentation
Org-act theory	Theory of hormonal organization and activation of brain structures mediating sex reflexes

PCOS	Polycystic ovary syndrome
Population frequency	Frequency in population, prevalence
Prenatal testosterone theory	Theory that level of prenatal testosterone is the mechanism causing TSTG
Puberty blocking	Prevention of puberty using hormones
Putamen	Brain structure mediating sensation and movement
Realization of TSTG	Awareness of TSTG starting at 4 years old
Reparative-like therapy	Therapy to eliminate TSTG
Reparative therapy	Therapy to change sexual orientation
SCID	Structured Clinical Interview for DSM
Sex	Sex organs
Sex organs	Biological organs enabling reproduction
Sexual arousal	Physiological preparation for sexual behavior
Sexual dimorphic structures	Anatomical structures that differ between males and females
Sexual fetish	Obtaining sexual arousal from nonhuman stimuli
Sexual orientation	Attraction and sexual arousal to particular sex
Social transition	Childhood full-time behavior according to congruent gender behavior category
Stealth	Transsexual living in secrecy
Top surgery	Mastectomy
Tranny	Pejorative for transsexual or transgender
Transgender	Phenomenon in which gender behavior or verbal declaration of gender identity is incongruent with assigned natal gender behavior category and congruent with some other gender behavior category
Transman	FTM transsexual or transgender person
Transsexual	Long-term transgender behavior with body change
Transvestite	Pejorative historical term for transgender
Transwoman	MTF transsexual or transgender person
TS genital plastic surgery	Culminating procedure for TS transition; also called as misnomers: gender reassignment

	surgery, gender confirmation surgery and sex-change surgery
TSTG	Transsexualism and transgenderism
Two-factor theory	Theory that genetics and epigenetics are causal factors in TSTG
Two-spirit	Native American gender-flexible people
Ventral tegmental area	Brain area providing dopamine to structures that mediate reward and addiction
Waria	Indonesian gender behavior category
White matter	Brain structures primarily containing neuronal connective tissue (axons)
Winkte	Lakota gender behavior category
WPATH	World Professional Association for Transgender Health
Xanith	Oman gender behavior category

1

Introduction

A TYPICAL TRANSGENDER STORY

An overnight snowfall had crippled transportation in the Northeast. All schools and businesses were closed on that January day in 1984. The snow continued. John and Jane, a married couple, watched the snow forecast on early morning television, and decided to go back to bed. Their bodies entwined to share their warmth. One thing led to another . . .

The child grew rapidly within Jane's womb, although she was initially unaware of its presence. After six weeks passed, Jane discovered that she had missed her period and went to see her doctor. He confirmed she was pregnant. Jane announced the news to John, and they both were joyful.

The pregnancy progressed without problem, except for a few days when Jane had flu-like symptoms, but she had been vaccinated against the flu shortly after learning of her pregnancy. The delivery was easy, and John and Jane felt happy to have a boy, whom they named William. William met all of his developmental milestones as expected and loved to play with his toy trucks and trains. By age 4, he was also becoming an early reader and showing that he preferred using his left hand for most tasks.

While William was growing up, John's and Jane's careers both took off. They were the best programmers in their company and received big promotions and raises. They were confident in their economic circumstances.

When William was old enough to walk, he would go into his parents' room and play with their drawer contents, clothes, shoes, and toiletries. John and

Jane thought that William's behavior was cute and did not think anything was wrong at first. But William gradually started playing exclusively with his mother's things. At William's fourth birthday party, he insisted on getting a pink party hat and pink party favor, even when both blue and pink were available.

A few months later he told his mother that he was a girl, not a boy.

Jane assured him that he was indeed a boy and would grow up to be just like his father. Jane did not think that William was serious about wanting to be a girl. However, a few weeks later, Jane found William with lipstick and her makeup on his face, wearing her panties. Jane helped him scrub the makeup off and change clothes, and she began to worry. William again told his mother that he knew that he was a boy but he wanted to be a girl, just like her. When John came home, Jane told him what had happened, and they both began to feel panic. They called their parents, who assured them that William was just going through a phase and it wouldn't last. After all, Jane had been a tomboy in her childhood and had "outgrown it."

William started kindergarten and did well until he got into conflict with his teacher. The teacher had instructed the class that the girls should go play in the section of the playroom with play kitchen, laundry, dining room, and feminine clothing. The boys had been told to go to the section with the play trucks, cowboy outfits, and a mock airplane that was big enough for one boy to sit in. William tried to go with the group of girls, but they reported him to the teacher. The teacher told him that he was not allowed to go with the girls or play in the girls' area. He temporarily went with the boys but snuck back to play in the girls' section. When the teacher discovered this, William was given a timeout of 5 minutes in the corner. During the next school day, events repeated themselves. The conflict with the teacher culminated in William having a temper tantrum. William lay on his back and banged his arms and legs on the floor. William's behavior triggered an immediate phone call by the teacher to Jane and John. The teacher insisted that they immediately leave work and come get their son. William was in big trouble.

John and Jane had a sit-down with William. He was told that he was embarrassing himself, his family, and his church by insisting that he wanted to be a girl. They insisted that he would grow up to be like his father and he would be responsible for having a family as a man. He was not to play with the girls. He was not to wear his mother's clothing and makeup. William was grounded for a week, and there were threats of spankings. During this session of reprimand, William cried, but he got the message, just not the message his parents intended.

William got the message that it was not safe for him to behave like a girl, even though he wanted to. He decided that he would stop talking about being a girl to his parents, and others, and just be a girl in private. He could sneak into his mother's room and borrow her clothing. He now knew how to take off makeup with tissue and makeup remover. He could now put on makeup and quickly take it off when he was in the locked bathroom. He would play along in school and at church. He would keep his secret from everyone. William was now a transgender child in the closet.

William grew into a teenager and young adult and played sports for the boys' teams. Although he did not particularly like his male body, it was fun to "take it out for a spin" to see what being a boy was like. Besides, no one would suspect what William did in private. And William had other good reasons to cross-dress in secret. He could see how boys who looked feminine or behaved in a feminine manner were bullied and attacked. He learned how to pretend to be masculine in public by carefully studying boy behavior. From all outward appearances and his sports involvement, it seemed that he was a well-adjusted all-American boy.

William soon became old enough to hang out with the girls. People regarded this as normal flirtation. He enjoyed the company of girls but had an additional motive, that of learning about feminine clothing and presentation through careful study of girls' behavior. William sometimes became uncomfortable with the girls because his male body sometimes responded by sexual arousal and an erection. He was expected to date girls, but during these dates would always wonder what he would do as the girl. To show his manhood, he sometimes aggressively pursued sex, but his heart was not in it, and he was not very successful.

When William finished school, he got a job and moved into an apartment. The apartment was small, but it gave him absolute privacy. For the first time he was able to dress from head to toe as a woman. He would come home, have dinner, and get cross-dressed. He then would watch television or go online on the Internet to chat with his transgender friends. William did this several times a week. At the beginning of these dress-up sessions, William would get erect because women's clothes felt and looked so different from men's clothes. At the end of the evening, he would shower and scrub off the makeup. While he scrubbed, William would masturbate, as he normally did in the shower.

To placate the men in the office, William would go on occasional dates, so that he could join discussions about their love lives. At work, he became as good a computer programmer as his parents had been and specialized in dealing with code that other programmers found impossible to fix.

After months of nightly dressing in his apartment, William went out in public as Billie for the first time. He was uncertain about doing this, but one of his online friends encouraged him to go to the local transgender support group. It provided a safe environment where Billie could cross-dress and the chance to meet some of his transgender online friends in person. Some attendees even dressed at the support group location to avoid leaving their homes cross-dressed.

Support group procedure was always the same. First an opportunity was given for people to stand up and identify themselves, or at least provide an alias. Next the support group would have a presentation, for example, wig-fitting and care. This was followed by group discussion. After the meeting, many members of the group went to a local nightclub that was transgender-friendly. The club even had restrooms for male, female, and "others." William became a regular at that bar and other transgender-friendly bars in the area.

Then William met Linda at work and fell in love. He felt close to her, and they had similar interests. He was lonely in his bachelor existence. The sex was good and Linda was understanding and enthusiastic. Although his online friends advised caution, William decided that it was time for him to settle down. He proposed marriage. William thought getting married would make him stop his cross-dressing.

After the honeymoon, William moved into Linda's apartment. Because he could not take his stash of feminine clothing and makeup with him to her apartment, he donated the clothing to Goodwill and threw away the makeup. He hoped that he would not need those items anymore.

The newlyweds adjusted to living together. But after 3 months, William found he still had the desire to cross-dress. After 2 more months of fighting the desire, he started to rummage through his wife's lingerie drawer and closet and found that they were about the same size. William started wearing his wife's panties to work, being careful to take them off in private when he got home. Whenever he thought he could safely do so, he tried on one of her dresses and applied makeup, followed by the usual scrubbing in the shower with masturbation. The couple soon found that they had sex less often, and occasionally William could not stay erect, usually within a few hours of his masturbation sessions. Linda was understanding; she figured the sexual cooling was normal because they were married. He was well practiced in secrecy, and William managed to keep his transgender secret from his wife and the people in his office, but he had to create excuses for the time he spent cross-dressing.

William's career was taking off. He became the designated "code fixer" for the company. This required visiting customer facilities in other cities for a few days at a time. William started cross-dressing on these trips. At first, he would put some of his wife's clothes into his suitcase, but later he started buying his own feminine clothing. He kept a bag loaded with Billie's clothing in the garage, so that it could easily be loaded into the car before he left for the airport. William soon outgrew a single bag and rented a small storage space, outfitting it with a cheap wardrobe closet.

William became a visiting member of support groups in Washington and Boston. He soon learned where all the transgender-friendly public places were in those cities, and extended his travel time into the weekend at least once a month. William was now living two separate lives, one at home and one on the road. He sometimes became panicky and depressed about his secret life as Billie and would "purge," or throw away, his Billie suitcase on his return trips.

He would feel safe for a month or so; then he would buy another suitcase and become Billie again while on the road. The cycle repeated itself several times. While all of this was going on, William and Linda had a child.

William had a severe automobile accident and had time to think while recovering in the hospital. He realized that life was too short to be isolated from others, especially his wife. He realized that the secret of his cross-dressing was beginning to interfere with his relationship with his wife. He felt guilty that he was deceiving her. He sat down with Linda and told her about Billie. Linda was confused and scared. Her feelings included sympathy for her spouse, anger at his deceptions, and doubt about her own sexuality. She was considering a divorce. Linda went to "significant other" (SO) meetings at the local transgender support group to understand her husband's behavior. She even attended a transgender convention in Atlanta that had a series of presentations and workshops for SOs while William attended the convention in full Billie mode.

Linda went through more periods of confusion and panic, wondering whether William would become a transsexual. William could not totally comfort her because he did not know what was happening to him either. William and Linda stayed together because they still loved each other and their child but remained uncertain about the future. William went to the local support group, instead of those out of town, and associated with his transgender friends with his wife's knowledge.

This is a typical transgender story, but this story also has a scientific explanation that will help in understanding transgender people and transsexuals. William's story will be retold in Chapter 14—this time with the omitted events that may have scientific meaning as described in Chapters 2 through 13.

UNDERSTANDING TRANSSEXUALISM AND TRANSGENDERISM

Science is beginning to help us understand transsexualism and transgenderism (TSTG), and promises to continue to improve our understanding in the future. Until the middle of the 20th century, the only information that was available about TSTG came from the clinical impressions and theories of mental health practitioners. Mental health professionals did their best to help transsexuals and transgendered people, and continue to do so. Although TSTG is no longer regarded as a disorder by most mental health professionals, transsexuals and transgender people still need help from mental health practitioners, as well as medical professionals, to help them deal with problems they face. There now exists scientific evidence that can help us understand TSTG and can guide evidence-based treatment.

Transsexualism and transgenderism is the result of a mismatch between biological gender predisposition and a person's culturally assigned gender behavior category. In most cultures, there are two gender behavior categories, masculine and feminine, but this is not universal. Biological gender predisposition results in behavioral tendencies. Culture creates gender behavior categories. In most cultures, a person's gender behavior category is usually determined based on assigned sex at birth or "natal sex." TSTG is a phenomenon in which the gender behavior or verbal declaration of gender identity of an individual is incongruent with their assigned natal gender behavior category, and congruent with some other gender behavior category. Until we have enough scientific evidence to separate them, transsexualism and transgenderism can be regarded as a singular behavioral phenomenon, differing only in frequency and degree of voluntary body change.

TSTG can now be regarded as a naturally occurring biological phenomenon. TSTG is part of the diversity of nature that allows our species to adapt to new environments. Biological causal factors have been identified and lower-level mechanisms can now be hypothesized for future scientific research.

The reason that scientific evidence is now available to help understand TSTG is the revolution in scientific instrumentation and measurement, primarily developed for improving medical science. An example is the development of genetic tools, during the international Human Genome Project, to understand DNA and how its information is expressed in human development and functioning. It is now possible to look for genetic differences between those with and those without TSTG. Another example is the development of brain imaging technologies, including magnetic resonance imaging (MRI), which can provide information about brain anatomy in live, awake human beings. Another is functional magnetic resonance imaging (fMRI), which provides near real-time information about brain functioning. MRI and fMRI have allowed us to find not only anatomical but also functional differences in the active human brain that are attributable to TSTG.

The revolution in scientific brain instrumentation will continue, and it is expected that our scientific knowledge of TSTG will grow as well. Current and future science can help us to understand TSTG more fully. For example, new brain imaging and measurement technologies are being developed, such as diffusion tensor imaging magnetic resonance imaging (DTI-MRI), that allow investigators to observe new types of brain phenomena in real time. Differences in microstructure that are attributable to TSTG have already been found using DTI. Advanced programs are now under way to model the brain and nervous system in computer systems to organize all the current and future scientific information.

However, current scientific knowledge and research of TSTG is spread across at least 22 scientific disciplines. Comprehensive understanding of TSTG requires that this information be identified, organized, and integrated. The logical scientific discipline to pull all this together is biopsychology because it focuses on how the brain generates behavior based on multiple scientific approaches. It is especially important to understand the current scientific evidence to identify directions for future research based on previous results because funding is limited. Research funding is typically directed toward treatments or cures for diseases and illnesses. TSTG is neither a disease nor an illness, so it is a low-priority area of research among government funding agencies. TSTG by definition violates cultural rules, and thus research is also underfunded because TSTG is rejected by those who regard current cultural rules as sacrosanct.

This book provides a snapshot of current scientific knowledge that helps us to understand TSTG. This first snapshot is intended to capture the fundamentals of TSTG science. The fine-grain detail will undoubtedly change in the future.

From a wide variety of medical, sociological, and psychological sources, Chapter 2 reviews the importance of TSTG not only to the individual but also to cultures at large. Both TSTG people and all of society bear financial and human costs because essential services are not provided to transsexual and transgender people and because their human and political rights are frequently denied.

Chapter 3 provides definitions of terms. Understanding any behavioral phenomenon requires carefully crafted definitions to minimize subjectivity. Relying on the tradition of the science of biopsychology, the goal in this chapter is to develop precise behavioral and objective definitions that can be applied to evidence across all scientific disciplines. The definitions assume that gender behavior categories are created by cultures and that TSTG behavior occurs when a person's assigned gender behavior category is incongruent with their biological gender predisposition. It is clear that gender behavior categories are created by culture because they vary from culture to culture both historically and geographically as indicated by evidence cited in Chapter 4. The transsexual or transgender person then seeks to follow another available gender behavior category. The terms *sex* and *gender* are not the same thing and should not be conflated.

Chapter 3 also provides information on the population frequencies of TSTG. This is an issue that bears on data interpretation for many of the relevant scientific disciplines because numerous research studies compare the frequencies observed in small clinical populations to those of the general population. The first, and still the best, population estimates of male-to-female TSTG were made by engineers using applied mathematical estimation theory, rather than counting patients coming through clinic doors. These estimates have increasingly been supported by recent psychological surveys. As a result of this analysis, the recent population estimates appear to be several orders of magnitude higher than previously thought.

Chapter 4 deals with anthropological and sociological evidence regarding TSTG. Many cultures rely on a binary gender system in which there are only two gender behavior categories, but there are other cultures that use multiple (three to five) gender behavior categories. Presumably these multiple categories evolved to accommodate the gender predisposition of offspring and organize an efficient division of labor. The diversity of cultures with multiple behavioral categories, both historically and geographically, supports the idea that gender predisposition and resulting TSTG originate from biological causal factors. Some cultures allow movement between gender behavior categories, for example those Native American tribes that recognized the "two-spirit" tradition. Some cultures do not tolerate movement between gender behavior categories.

Evidence for a genetic causal factor is reviewed in Chapter 5. Scientific evidence from genetics reveals that human DNA plays a strong role as a causal factor in TSTG and in forming human gender behavior predisposition. Because TSTG begins to be realized at or near age 4, genetics is one of the few candidate factors that could influence behavior early in development. Heritability studies involving identical twins and families indicate significant loadings for a genetic factor in TSTG. If one identical twin is transsexual or transgender, then it is more likely the other twin will also be TSTG than the population frequencies. Furthermore, DNA markers have been found for TSTG. Significant differences between TSTG and non-TSTG can also be found in genetic biomarkers, although a full DNA scan has not yet been performed. Taken together, the evidence indicates that genetics are a significant causal factor for TSTG.

The new science of epigenetics is important for an understanding of TSTG, as described in Chapter 6. Epigenetics involves the study of mechanisms that modify DNA, or change its expression, and thus shape the body and behavior of a person. Epigenetics combines genetics, pharmacology, toxicology, and physiology and other sciences. Epigenetics is another candidate biological causal factor for TSTG because it begins before conception and continues through the childhood period before TSTG begins to be realized. Most epigenetic mechanisms begin at conception, but some actually start before conception. Epigenetics fits with the timing of the early emergence of TSTG, which is consistent with epigenetics being a candidate causal factor. There is evidence that this causal factor may correlate with TSTG. The evidence supporting an epigenetic factor is positive, but limited. Prenatal exposure to drugs, toxic chemicals, and prenatal stress can cause mutations or change DNA expression. There are myriad potential epigenetic mechanisms for causation of TSTG. The most exciting are the recently discovered epigenetic mechanisms that involve the exchange of cells and chemicals between mother and fetus. Just as the entire DNA can now be scanned to look for TSTG DNA markers, it is now possible to perform a scan that indicates the influence of epigenetic modifications to DNA that change DNA expression. Epigenetics represents a viable second causal factor in TSTG. However, this evidence is only suggestive that future research should be pursued.

The two-factor theory of TSTG causation is presented in Chapter 7. This theory is an attempt to integrate genetic and epigenetic factors that form the biological basis for TSTG. There are many examples of phenomena that also have genetics and epigenetics as causal factors. One of these phenomena is handedness. Handedness refers to the preference of right or left hand for various tasks. It is significant that transsexuals tend to be less right-handed than nontranssexuals. The evidence for the two-factor theory explains the interplay between genetics and epigenetics in TSTG.

Chapter 8 helps us understand that the behavior of parents toward their children is not a causal factor in TSTG. Child rearing and parent-child interaction are explored causal factors for TSTG because they start in early childhood. However, evidence from developmental child psychology studies does not support these potential causal factors. Some transsexual and transgender children, like William, seeing that they will face rejection if their behavior breaches cultural norms, adopt a strategy of secrecy in childhood. They keep their TSTG behavior secret from their parents and family. Other children, despite cultural rejection, attempt a social transition in childhood, and some seek out drugs to block puberty. Delaying puberty gives the children more time to decide whether to begin transsexual transition using cross-sex hormones at age 16 or later. Although child rearing and parental interactions do not seem to cause TSTG, parental reaction should be guided by understanding, not culturally supported prejudice.

Chapter 9 deals with the formation of sexual arousal and TSTG behavior during the period of adolescence and young adulthood. Sexual arousal is actually a learned phenomenon that involves classical conditioning, sometimes called Pavlovian conditioning. Classical conditioning theory also predicts the extinction of learned responses with repeated unreinforced exposure to the eliciting stimuli. TSTG behavior persists even after extinction of learned sexual arousal responses to opposite-gender clothing and presentation, indicating that sexual arousal and fetishism are not causal factors in TSTG. Surveys of transgender people also indicate that they cross-dress for relaxation not for fetishism. A behavioral psychology taxonomy is proposed to organize gender tasks and provide a tool for understanding cultural differences regarding TSTG over time and space. During the period of adolescence and young adulthood, all people, including nontranssexual and nontransgender people, learn about sexual arousal through emotional systems in the brain and also learn about appropriate behavior for gender behavior categories.

Chapter 10 presents the relatively recent evidence that TSTG is correlated with differences in neuroanatomy and neurophysiological function. The evidence includes neuroanatomical differences, differences detected by MRI, and differences in neurophysiology detected by fMRI. These differences provide further support for the idea that TSTG have a biological basis.

Chapter 11 deals with the issue of what triggers TSTG behavior, and whether TSTG behavior is a conscious lifestyle choice, and how the experience of gendered spirituality is mediated by the brain. Transsexuals and transgender people sometimes suddenly increase their TSTG behavior due to personal loss or changes in life circumstances. This phenomenon is explained by reference to a clinical counseling technique that provokes "existential crises" in patients to change their behavior. Biopsychology provides some understanding as to whether TSTG is a conscious lifestyle choice or a biological imperative. In this case, cognitive neuroscience has provided information. The biological imperative wins out because there is no such thing as a conscious choice. Cognitive neuroscience evidence indicates that humans are only conscious of choices well after they are made by subconscious mechanisms. Historically, and even today, there are members of North American native tribes who claim that they experience inspiration from two genders. If these "two-spirit" individuals experience two gender manifestations of spirituality, how then does the brain mediate these experiences? We cannot deny the experience of spirituality, which is profound for many human beings, but we can conclude that there is no proof that there are interfaces between ethereal spirits and the brain. Indeed, the idea that ethereal spirits interact with the brain to cause behavior contradicts the definition of both ethereal spirits and corporeal biology. Subconscious mechanisms appear to mediate both choice and the experience of spirituality. Two-spirits are likely to have two subconscious biological gender predispositions.

Chapter 12 presents historical information about psychodynamic theories of TSTG and about the insurance coding conventions regarding TSTG provided by the *Diagnostic and Statistical Manual* (5th edition; DSM-V) and 10th and 11th versions of the *International Classification of Diseases* (ICD-10 and ICD-11). Changes to these coding schemes have become an objective in the depathologization of TSTG. Psychodynamic theories do not constitute scientific theories because they lack scientific rigor. They cannot be reduced to practice to allow experimentation and testing. Scientific theories must make clear predictions of experimental results. Psychodynamic theories are often used, and sometimes misconstrued, to indicate that transsexualism and transgenderism are pathological.

The DSM of the American Psychiatric Association is the reference that currently codifies mental illnesses in the United States for insurance purposes. In the recent version, DSM-V, the TSTG category of gender identity disorder was taken out of its previous mental disorder category in an effort to depathologize it.

The DSM-V also continues to include transvestic fetishism and autogynephilia as causes of TSTG that provides the basis for pathologization of TSTG by opponents. WPATH has objected to the continuation of autogynephilia because it is unproven.

Chapter 13 covers transsexual transition procedures for body modification. The goal of transition is to make sex organs look more male or more female and help bring TSTG presentation into alignment with cultural expectations of the congruent gender behavior category of a transsexual. Some nontranssexual transgender people also undergo these procedures. There is a strong drive for body change among transsexuals, and some transgender people, that is expressed by taking cross-sex hormones and undergoing surgeries and other procedures. Transsexual transition typically involves the cooperation of mental health, endocrinology, and medical professionals. Transsexual transition does involve some medical risks, but medical, mental health professionals, and transsexuals consider these risks to be offset by the positive effects. Transition greatly helps transsexuals, and most are satisfied with the results. Some transsexuals have verbally expressed regret, but they are few in number. Many transsexuals change their sexual orientation during or after transition. Understanding transsexual transition helps us understand that medical authorities, as well as TSTG, regard transition as a necessity, and demonstrates the commitment of transsexuals to live in a more congruent gender behavior category.

Chapter 14 provides a conclusion to the book that includes the full story of William and summarizes what we now know about TSTG from scientific evidence.

Also provided in this book are suggestions for further reading (Appendix A) and a listing of organizations serving the transsexual and transgender community (Appendix B).

Why Understanding Transsexualism and Transgenderism Is Important

2.0 INTRODUCTION

Why do you need to understand transsexualism and transgenderism (TSTG)? The short answer is that both individuals and governments pay high human and economic costs for rejecting transsexuals and transgender individuals. Improved understanding of the TSTG phenomenon should help reduce rejection and the consequences of rejection (definition of TSTG is provided in Section 3.1.1). Understanding TSTG is important and requires an appreciation of the negative consequences that both the individual and cultures experience as a result of collisions between TSTG gender behavior predisposition and culturally established gender behavior categories.

By definition, TSTG is a behavioral violation of culture rules and norms regarding gender behavior categories (see Section 3.1.1.4 for definition). For this reason, TSTG behavior is typically rejected by cultures at the individual, family, community, and institutional levels. At the individual level, TSTG behavior may result in slurs, microaggressions, bullying, or violence. TSTG behavior may result in ejection from the family. Rejection of TSTG occurs in many ways by many sources, all of which contribute to the human and economic costs.

As an ethical and practical matter, governments should attempt to reduce the suffering of the human beings within their domains, including transsexuals and transgender people. For example, the attempted suicide rate among transsexuals and transgender people is in the range of 31% to 43% (Bauer, Pyne, Fancion,

& Hammond, 2013; Grant et al., 2010; Liu & Mustanski, 2001; Mustanski & Liu, 2010, 2013). The high suicide rate results in unnecessary suffering by transsexuals, transgender people, and those who love them. The high rate also results in emergency room and mental health costs, which the government and its citizens end up paying directly or indirectly. The suicide rate could be reduced by more effective TSTG mental health and social services. Another example is the unfair treatment of transsexual and transgender employees by companies and governments. The result of the suffering this causes is that employers lose large amounts of money in the form of time lost, loss of productivity, attempted suicide, and poor reputation as a result of poor employee treatment. Governments often do not provide workplace protections or interpret labor standards to protect TSTG. Many transsexual and transgender children are made homeless by their families and communities and end up in the street engaging in the sex trade. This creates a reservoir of venereal diseases including HIV infection. If communities want to deal with these public health issues, they need to start by understanding that transsexuals and transgender people are on the street not because they want to be there but because they have few other options. Those cities that understand this TSTG problem have started diversion programs to find jobs and housing for those picked up for street crime rather than incarcerating them. Many companies and governments who understand TSTG have set up mechanisms to reduce the human and economic costs.

This chapter describes some of the many ways in which transsexuals and transgender people are rejected by their cultures and the resulting costs. Many people need this information, not the least of which are transsexuals and transgender people themselves. It is also important for medical and mental health professionals who encounter TSTG patients. It is important for teachers who must deal with students as they mature. It is important for journalists, government officials, and others in the public sphere to advocate policy based on factual evidence as it relates to the TSTG phenomena. It is important for them to learn about the situation in which transsexuals and transgender people find themselves to develop public understanding. Rather than succumbing to fear and hysteria, governmental personnel need to understand the ways that TSTG creates rejection so that public health and other policies are based on facts about TSTG. For the general public, understanding of TSTG science is important because we are continuously exposed to pseudoscience and hate mongering in the media.

This chapter provides an overview of the ways in which transsexuals and transgender people are rejected and the associated costs. Some of the human and cultural costs are listed in Table 2.1 and each of them will be described in this chapter.

Table 2.1. Human and cultural costs of rejecting transsexuals and transgender people

Cost Factor	Human	Culture
Secrecy	High mental workload	Reduced productivity
	Loneliness	Reduced productivity
	Loss of authenticity	Reduced productivity
	Depression	Depression medication and mental health costs
	Suicide attempts	Emergency department subsidies
	Suicides	Labor force loss
Homelessness		
	Ill health	TSTG housing program costs
	Poverty	Social services costs
	Prostitution	STD/HIV reservoir
	Drug addiction	Drug trade
School		
	High mental workload	Wasted instructional costs
	Loss of authenticity	Loss of creativity
	Bullying and harassment	Bullying program costs; lost instruction time
	Traumatic injury	Emergency department subsidies and medical insurance costs
	Inappropriate restroom assignment	Litigation costs
Health care		
	Rejection by medical personnel	Increased medical insurance costs
	Inability to get appropriate medical insurance	Emergency department subsidies
	Inappropriate treatment	Litigation costs
	Inappropriate mental health treatment	Attempted suicide costs
		Additional medical costs
Job Discrimination		
	Job and promotion discrimination	Reduced access to talent

(Continued)

Table 2.1. *(Continued)*

Cost Factor	Human	Culture
	Bullying and harassment	Bullying program costs; reduced productivity
	Inability to transfer to other countries/ locations	Reduced business personnel transfer flexibility
	Inappropriate restroom assignment	Litigation costs; lost work time
Discriminatory Laws		
	Unnecessary surgeries required for changing ID marker	Increased medical costs
	Death or imprisonment in some countries	Reduced business personnel transfer flexibility
Public Accommodations		
	Public harassment	Increased potential for violence
	Rejection by businesses	Loss of revenue
	Rejection or sexual harassment by police	Litigation costs
Legal Identification		
	Unnecessary surgeries for birth certificate change	Increased medical costs
	Amending vs. reissue with new gender marker	Job discrimination
	Refusal/difficulty to get driver's license	Loss of DMV time and voting discrimination
Incarceration		
	Denial of hormones and surgeries	Attempted suicide costs
	Physical assault if inappropriate incarceration assignment	Medical costs

Table 2.1. *(Continued)*

Cost Factor	Human	Culture
Self-understanding		
	Inability to train inexperienced medical providers	Litigation costs
	Loss of peace of mind and increased mental workload	Loss of productivity and creativity
Military Service		
	Inability to serve their country	Military labor force loss of motivated people
	Costs of secrecy for those in service	

2.1 COSTS OF SECRECY

To avoid rejection, many transsexuals and transgender people become secretive about their gender behavior category expression. In reaction to rejection and anticipated rejection, most transsexuals and transgender children resort to secrecy at an early age. The realization that one is transsexual or transgender typically occurs at age 3 to 5 years, after one has gained a familiarity with gender behavior categories at 2 to 3 years of age (Kennedy & Helen, 2010). It may begin with discouraging comments or punishment by parents, family, or people in the community. Typical early TSTG behaviors include playing with cosmetics or wearing mother's clothing by male-to-female transgender children or wearing pants and refusing to wear dresses by female-to-male transgender children.

Cross-dressing behavior typically starts with only a few items but typically develops into complete cross-gender presentation in private and eventually in public. Many adult transsexuals and transgender people feel the need to go to support groups or bars where they might be accepted in public, but they do so undercover with assumed names and identities. This is the "standard operating procedure" of many transgender people who periodically dress and go out while continuing their secrecy. Transgender people are able to balance work and family with gender behavior category expression.

Most transsexual and transgender individuals do not seek mental health treatment because they want to maintain secrecy. They feel no need for treatment and consequently are not included in clinical statistics. This is particularly true if they are in military or other occupations in which TSTG behavior is grounds for dismissal or loss of security clearances. Surprisingly, transgender people are twice as likely as nontransgender people to join the military, as described in Section 9.8. Secrecy starts at an early age and may continue in different forms. Now that the U.S. military Don't Ask, Don't Tell law has been repealed, there is a movement to allow transgender people to serve openly. This would not require a change in the law, only a change in military medical policy.

Because of increasing understanding of TSTG, it is now possible for many transsexual and transgender children to live openly in the opposite gender behavior category, block puberty with hormones, and eventually decide whether to transition after age 16 to 18. This minimizes the secrecy period except for the period before age 16, when they are in school and do not have appropriate legal gender status. We discuss these new procedures more fully in Chapters 8 and 9.

Some transsexual and transgender people decide that they want voluntary body changes and start transsexual transition procedures (Chapter 13). After completing transition, a transsexual may go back into secrecy, termed *living in stealth*, in which they change names, locations, and friends to establish new identities, with the goal of avoiding suspicion of their history. If they are successful, they may disappear from TSTG statistics altogether. Living in stealth is controversial because other transsexuals and transgender people feel that they have been abandoned by their transsexual friends who have gone into stealth. By living in stealth, transsexuals are also not in position to advocate for granting transsexual and transgender people their rights. Living in stealth is yet another form of TSTG secrecy.

There is a body of psychological science that examines the potential adverse effects of secrecy (Kelly, 2002). This science indicates that those protecting a secret must constantly calculate how to lie and maneuver to avoid discovery. This requires a highly stressful mental workload that interferes with vocational and avocational productivity. When a transsexual or transgender person is asked at work about what he or she did the previous weekend, they have to have cover stories ready to avoid talking about going to a TSTG convention or clubbing with their transsexual and transgender friends. More than 70% of transsexuals and transgender people report hiding their TSTG at work (Grant et al., 2010). At home after a business trip, transsexuals and transgender people have to lie to provide a convincing story for their families. Even simple intellectual tasks become stressful, such as using the right gender pronoun or correct proper name. All this lying and calculation becomes mentally exhausting. Because secrecy is toxic, the potential adverse effects of secrecy may spread to wives and significant others if they also attempt to maintain the secrets.

In addition to the adverse physical and mental effects caused by secrecy, many experience loss of authenticity (Kelly, 2002) through the process of constantly denying their sense of who they really are with regard to their gender predisposition. They may repeatedly hear or see themselves reject TSTG and even join in group harassment of other transsexuals and transgender people when they, themselves, are not cross-dressed. Authenticity is essential to well-being, both psychologically (Wood, Linley, Maltby, Baliousis, & Joseph, 2008) and physically (Kelly, 2002).

Secrecy brings with it loss of self-esteem and the suffering of physical stress, isolation, loneliness, depression, and often suicide. Physical stress causes medical problems and weakened immune response. Many transsexuals and transgender people avoid other people and choose loneliness to avoid revealing their secrets during any close personal relationships. Avoidance of others contributes to depression. The consequent rate of depression in TSTG individuals has been assessed at more than 60% (Rotondi et al., 2011). Secrecy leads to mental effects that in turn have physical consequences.

Secrecy takes its toll on authenticity and creates depression and loneliness, but it also triggers suicide and contributes to the high suicide rate among young adults. The frequency of attempted suicide in transsexuals and transgender people is believed to be approximately 31% to 43% (Bauer, Pyne, Fancion, & Hammond, 2013; Grant et al., 2010; Liu & Mustanski, 2001; Mustanski & Liu, 2010, 2013), as compared with the national frequency of 1.6%. Some suicides can be confirmed from evidence left behind, but many suicides due to TSTG rejection probably go undetected. The rate of attempted suicides among transsexual and transgender people undoubtedly contributes to the overall high suicide rate in young people.

Transsexuals and transgender individuals who attempt suicide have 10 times greater odds of a reattempt within a year (Mustanski & Liu, 2013). Surveys of transsexual and transgender people indicate that two of every three have contemplated suicide in their lives (Testa et al., 2012). Transsexual suicide attempts are sometimes provoked by the inability to obtain breast implants or other surgeries. Transsexuals are often unable to obtain such surgeries because of the financial burden and because of delays in government health services. TSTG does not go away and continues to trigger suicide attempts into adulthood.

The high rate of depression and attempted suicide among transsexual and transgender individuals means that governments and other institutions need to establish better youth mental health and suicide prevention programs aimed at the particular needs of this population. It also means that bullying of transsexual and transgender children and teens by students, teachers, and coworkers must be brought under control.

The effects of secrecy go well beyond an individual transsexual or transgender person to everyone that that person entrusts with the restricted information. The toxicity for these confidants includes the same phenomena as with the person who disclosed the secret. They must spend brain energy figuring out how to keep the secret, and they also lose their authenticity. Thus the toxic effects of secrecy extend beyond transsexual and transgender people to confidants, spouses, significant others, and friends.

TSTG secrecy has adverse health and productivity effects that need to be understood by both transsexuals and transgender people and cultures. The individual health effects include stress, depression, and potential suicide. Individual productivity effects stem from inauthenticity and the high mental workload necessary to maintain secrecy. Cultures are adversely affected by the health care costs resulting from depression and attempted suicide. Society is also affected by loss of productivity at work and in other activities due to inauthenticity.

2.2 HOMELESSNESS AND PROSTITUTION

Because of lack of understanding by cultures, transsexuals and transgender people, especially children, are prone to become homeless and to engage in a variety of street activities including prostitution, the drug trade, and drug use. More than 16% of transsexuals and transgender people report working in illegal street economies (Grant et al., 2011). Transsexuals and transgender individuals are not on the street because they want to be there; they are there because of rejection. The effects of homelessness and crime have a large impact on public health. Worldwide, transsexuals and transgender people on the street are 49 times as likely to have HIV (Baral et al., 2013) and are carriers of other venereal diseases. TSTG constitutes a huge public health problem by creating a reservoir for HIV and other venereal diseases (Clements-Nolle, Marx, Guzman, & Katz, 1991; Clements-Nolle, Wilkinson, & Kitano, 2001).

The root cause of homelessness and prostitution is the rejection of TSTG by family, church, social institutions, and governments (Bockting, Robinson, & Rosser, 1998; Boles & Elifson, 1994; Pang, Pugh, & Catalan, 1994; Clements-Nolle, Marx, & Katz, 2006; Quintana, Rosenthal, & Krehely, 2010). At least 57% of transsexuals and transgender individuals experience significant family rejection (Grant et al., 2010). To survive, homeless transsexuals and transgender people frequently participate in whatever street economic activity is available. Rejection is a result of the lack of understanding of the phenomena of TSTG. When many people see transsexual and transgender prostitutes in the street, they believe that they are there because they want to be there, but the fact is, they have nowhere else to go.

Many homeless shelters in the United States will not help a transsexual or transgender person unless they present in their culturally assigned gender behavior category (Bagby, 2013), particularly those associated with church organizations. At least one transgender death due to rejection by a homeless shelter has been documented, and there are undoubtedly others. In this case, the shelter was run by a religious organization (Wright, 2008). In many places, because of lack of understanding, no government or private social work programs are available to meet the needs of the TSTG population.

Transsexuals and transgender people experience discrimination in the workplace and are often unable to retain a job (Leichtentritt & Arad, 2004; Sausa, Keatley, & Operario, 2007), resulting in an unemployment rate of about 40% (Make the Road, 2010). Prostitution and drug-trade convictions and registry on the sex offender list ensure that some transsexuals and transgender people will have difficulty getting regular jobs. TSTG rejection leads to loss of charitable services and unemployment.

Transsexual and transgender people are disproportionately poor. Because of cultural rejection, they are four times more likely to have incomes under $10,000. Many leave or lose employment because of harassment on the job, and for those the rate of homelessness quadruples (Grant et al., 2010). The situation is even worse for TSTG of color (Grant et al., 2010).

Social work programs addressing the particular needs of street transsexuals or transgender people (Durso & Gates, 2012) could have a big payoff in terms of healthier lives (Spicer, 2010) and crime reduction. In particular, there are prostitution conviction diversion programs that defer prosecution of transsexuals or transgender individuals to allow for counseling, drug therapy, and job assistance. However, the success of such programs relies on an understanding of TSTG among the employees and other stakeholders of these social service agencies, which is currently lacking in many places. Some cities have established model programs that support housing and health needs, but many citizens and governmental officials regard TSTG problems as being due to a conscious lifestyle choice and should not be addressed. We examine the issue of conscious lifestyle choice in Chapter 11.

2.3 COSTS OF TSTG REJECTION AT SCHOOL

Because most societies require universal education, transsexual and transgender children must go to school or be homeschooled. As a reflection of cultural norms regarding gender behavior categorization, schools represent a danger zone. School is often the first sustained public performance for those who are presenting according to either congruent and incongruent gender behavior categories. The primary dangers for transsexuals and transgender people are bullying and violence. The rate of school harassment for transsexual and transgender individuals is estimated at 78%, the rate of physical assault is 35%, and the rate of sexual violence is 12% (Grant et al., 2011). It is the nature of school-age children that those students who show any deviation from gender behavior categories are identified for bullying and harassment. This comes at a time when the bullies themselves are still learning gender behavior rules. In their desire to express themselves, transsexuals and transgender children often run afoul of dress code or other regulations in school. Many of the most publicized legal cases involve extracurricular programs, such as proms and dances or public restroom policies.

Many transsexuals and transgender children successfully continue to employ secrecy in school to avoid confrontation as was described in Section 2.1. Some male-to-female transsexual and transgender children pursue all-male sports in an effort to "grow out" of their TSTG tendencies and/or to reduce suspicion. The aim of such efforts is similar to TSTG military and marriage flight that are discussed in Section 9.7. TSTG secrecy adds an additional burden to the stresses of going through childhood and adolescence.

Some transsexual and transgender children are only partially successful in using secrecy and are subjected to intense bullying and harassment in school. Because they are at variance with cultural norms, they are more susceptible than most of their peers. More than 51% of this population reports bullying in school (Grant et al., 2011). There is believed to be a direct connection among bullying, abuse, and harassment and transsexual/transgender attempted suicide (Clements-Nolle, Marx, & Kate 2006). This can occur at school—by both students and teachers (Kosciw, Greytak, Bartkiewicz, Boesen, & Palmer, 2012)—or on the street. Unfortunately, teachers also participate in harassment, and those who are abused by teachers are more likely to need long-term medical treatment. Because of this harassment, at least 15% of transsexuals and transgender children leave school during the K–12 years. Including school and elsewhere, more than 60% of this population experiences physical and sexual violence (Grant et al., 2010).

School officials, students, and the public have become aware of bullying and violence, largely due to cases of teen suicide resulting from bullying that have been publicized. Although some progress has been made through increased awareness, there are legal barriers to developing an understanding of GLBT from bans in some localities on discussion of GLBT issues in the schools. Understanding TSTG should assist in structuring school antibullying efforts by providing scientific facts to reduce prejudice (Kennedy, 2008).

Recently, there has been a movement for early recognition of transsexual and transgender children, allowing them to live according to their congruent gender behavior category starting in early childhood—termed *social transition*. Some even postpone puberty by using hormones to facilitate later transsexual transition. Stealth cannot typically be used to cover such behavior because birth certificates must be produced when starting school. This sets up potential conflicts with schools and states where gender behavior category rules do not allow such behavior.

Even if the school allows TSTG behavior, there is still the problem of sexually segregated facilities, especially restrooms and locker rooms. Most mental health professionals recommend that transsexual or transgender students use the facilities associated with their gender behavior category presentation. This is for the mental health of the student. However, some schools and states refuse to support restroom entry based on gender presentation. This results in ostracism and bullying. Some states, notably California, have passed laws requiring appropriate access for transsexual and transgender students; others have only legal precedents based on state constitutions.

The "restroom issue" continues to be battled out in U.S. politics as a social issue wedge that divides voters and raises money for advocacy institutions and hate mongers. Most mental health professionals advocate that use of the congruent restroom is necessary for the well-being of transsexual and transgender people. Those transsexuals who are engaged in their Real Life Experience procedure are expected to use their congruent restroom in order to complete the procedure (see Chapter 13). Those opposed to allowing transsexuals and transgender people access to their congruent gender behavior category facility maintain that it is dangerous to allow a transwoman to go into ladies' restrooms because she could attack females there. However, there are absolutely no confirmed incidents in which a male-to-female transsexual or transgender person actually attacked anyone in a ladies' restroom in the United States.

2.4 HEALTH CARE

Transsexual and transgender individuals have valid and unique health care issues that should be addressed by medical authorities, employers, and governments for both ethical and practical reasons. To address these needs, the people involved with these institutions need to understand the nature of TSTG (Gardner & Safer, 2013). In a recent survey, more than 50% of transsexual and transgender people said that they had to educate their medical provider on TSTG treatment (Grant et al., 2010). Medical schools in the United States and Canada currently provide approximately 5 hours of training on gay, lesbian, bisexual, and transgender (GLBT) medical issues that perforce includes little TSTG training (Obedin-Maliver et al., 2011). Professional medical societies and the U.S. National Institutes of Health encourage continuing education classes on TSTG cultural competency (Studwell, 2013). Understanding the nature of TSTG is gradually becoming a requirement for medical and mental health professionals.

Because transsexuals and transgender individuals are uniquely subject to violence at school, work, and in public, they often require medical treatment. More than 61% of TSTG report physical assaults, and 64% report sexual assault (Grant et al., 2011).

The first health care hurdle for transsexual and transgender people is to get treatment from a medical practitioner. The second hurdle is to get insurers to pay for it. In a national survey, 19% to 27% of transgender people reported being rejected for treatment because of prejudice by medical practitioners (Grant et al., 2010). Many more have had medical claims rejected because of gender marker mismatches for diagnostics or treatments—for example, male-to-female transsexuals and transgender people getting mammograms because they are on hormone therapy. This is despite guidelines from many medical certification authorities that indicate the need for serving the trans-sexual/transgender community. The Gay and Lesbian Medical Association (2014) provides a list of these guidelines for medical practitioners. The American College of Obstetricians and Gynecologists (2011) has issued guidelines for health care of transgender people. There are many reasons cited for rejection of treatment, and they all stem from a lack of understanding. These include violating cultural norms, lack of training on TSTG issues, lack of insurance coverage, and underestimation of the actual size of the TSTG population.

Mental health for transsexuals and transgender people should begin with reassurance and affirmation (Nuttbrook, Rosenblum, & Blumentstein, 2002) that their gender predisposition and behavior are nothing to worry about. Then they can be helped to deal with conflicts between their gender expression and culture. This is particularly true for children. Transsexuals and transgender people also need information on, for example, safe places to obtain the items and services needed for gender behavior category presentation.

Although reparative-like therapy for TSTG is banned in the United States by most mental health professional societies, the practice continues—notably with children. Reparative-like therapy includes a subset of the techniques ostensibly used to "cure" homosexuality. Reparative-like therapies include operant conditioning or pseudoscientific procedures to punish TSTG behavior and reward gender behavior in line with a person's culturally assigned sex. Reparative therapy has been demonstrated to be ineffective and to cause psychological harm. Such therapeutic attempts betray a fundamental lack of understanding of the inherent biological nature of TSTG among providers.

Because of job discrimination, many transsexuals and transgender people do not have health care coverage from their employers, and most policies have exceptions for TSTG treatment. Both the American Medical Association and the American Psychological Association have taken the position that treatment of TSTG is a medical necessity and should be included in health benefit plans. Medical insurance provided by employers has traditionally banned treatment for TSTG because insurers believed that it increased their financial risk. However, Fortune 1000 companies are increasingly providing TSTG treatment because they want to attract the best talent, they understand that transsexual and transgender people are valuable employees, and they understand that there is no increase in financial risk (as discussed later). The Human Rights Campaign (HRC) publishes a corporate equality index that includes information as to whether a corporation claims to provide TSTG specific health care. HRC found that 33% of businesses in their most recent survey provided some form of TSTG health care benefit. However, the HRC does not actually monitor the corporations for compliance or handle employee complaints.

Studies by the Williams Institute of 34 employers indicate that the cost of TSTG corporate health care coverage is low and does not increase insurers' overall financial risk (Herman, 2013). Experiences by government organizations including the City and County of San Francisco and the University of California confirm this conclusion. Coverage actually reduces other potential expensive risks that transsexuals and transgender people are prone to be subject to such as depression, medical treatment due to attempted suicide, and do-it-yourself hormone therapy gone wrong. In the United States, the Affordable Care Act and government regulation of health care have already provided additional benefits to transsexual and transgender people. For example, Medicare and the Veterans Health Administration (VHA Directive 2011-024) now cover diagnostic testing and hormones for transsexuals. Medicare provides coverage for transsexual genital plastic surgery but only in the five states that allow it. Whether competitive health care exchanges, VA, and Medicaid will cover TSTG-specific treatment such as genital plastic surgery and other surgeries is still under study.

Physicians need to be aware that transsexuals and transgender people have higher risk for certain medical illnesses than the general population (see Sections 13.2.1.2.2, 13.2.2.2.2, 13.4). The biggest risk for male-to-female transsexuals and transgender people is blood clots due to the estrogen they are taking in hormone therapy. Female-to-male transsexuals are particularly susceptible to polycystic ovary syndrome (PCOS) due to high testosterone levels before and after hormone therapy is begun.

2.5 WORKPLACE

The primary workplace concerns of TSTG are job discrimination, bullying/harassment, and restroom policy (Grant et al., 2011).

Most people would be surprised to learn that U.S. federal and most state laws provide no hiring/job discrimination protection for transsexual or transgender workers. Currently only 16 states provide employment discrimination protection (Transgender Law and Policy Institute, 2014) in the United States. More than 47% of transsexuals and transgender people report being fired from a job because of their status (Grant et al., 2011). As a result, there are numerous legal cases of hiring discrimination and unlawful discharge that generally rely on sexual discrimination statutes (Title VII of the Civil Rights Act). As a result of these cases and the most recent case *Macy v. Holder* the U.S. Equal Employment Opportunity Commission (EEOC) formally ruled that Title VII of the Civil Rights Act protects TSTG individuals from workplace discrimination. There will undoubtedly be more legal cases and further interpretations by the EEOC, but this was a landmark case for TSTG rights. Enforcement of this policy may still require costly legal suits. For that reason, there is no substitute for extension of workplace rights through laws such as the often-proposed U.S. Employment Non-Discrimination Act (ENDA). GLBT advocacy organizations have recently abandoned the 2014 draft ENDA version because it does not provide sufficient protection against religious discrimination in the wake of the outcome of the *Burwell v. Hobby Lobby* (formerly *Sebelius v. Hobby Lobby*) case. Market forces have encouraged more than 80% of the larger businesses on the HRC index to offer employment protection. TSTG still face workplace discrimination, but the trend is toward offering improved protections.

Transsexual and transgender people face verbal and physical harassment in their places of employment. In the workplace, 90% of TSTG report harassment as well as hiring and promotion discrimination (Grant et al., 2011). Just as it is clear that sexual harassment is banned by civil rights laws, the Macy case should now make it clear that TSTG harassment is also banned. But rulings by the EEOC are no substitute for employers being proactive to reduce harassment in the workplace.

Restrooms continue to be an issue in the workplace. Transsexuals and transgender workers are often required to walk longer distances than necessary to use family restrooms rather than use the bathroom associated with their congruent gender behavior category and presentation. Mental health authorities advocate that TSTG should use the restroom corresponding to their gender presentation. There are deleterious effects on the health of transsexual and transgender employees and the morale of a workplace related to this problem. Delaying use of restrooms can encourage urinary tract infections. However, where training for employees and managers is provided to understand TSTG issues, restroom problems can usually be resolved.

2.6 DISCRIMINATORY LAWS

Transsexuals and transgender people face capital punishment, imprisonment, and fines in many countries outside of the United States. These laws exist despite United Nations activity aimed at securing TSTG rights in all countries. The European Union has made progress in reducing TSTG discrimination, but it still continues (Amnesty International, 2014). Discriminatory countries are located primarily in North Africa and the Middle East. The rationale for these foreign laws is that TSTG is unnatural and can be cured by reparative-like therapy. Unethical groups from the United States and elsewhere urged these countries to adopt such discriminatory laws, but they now deny such advocacy. They have provided misinformation regarding reparative therapy in an attempt to convince lawmakers that TSTG is a conscious lifestyle choice that can be changed. Advocacy by these groups for reparative therapy continues, even though it is repudiated by professional mental health organizations in the United States and illegal in many states and countries. Such therapy is ineffective and injurious to the subject of the therapy.

Iran is an interesting case in which GLB activities bring a death sentence, but transsexuals are treated somewhat differently. Because of a religious *fatwa* by the Ayatollah Khomeini, transsexuals are exempt from the capital punishment law if they have had TS genital plastic surgery (GPS); sometimes referred to as "sex change" surgery. Iranian transsexuals are encouraged to get TS GPS as soon as possible, and there are medical subsidies provided by the government. Those transsexuals who do not want GPS fall into the same category as GLB people and are vulnerable to capital punishment. The result is that Iran purportedly performs more TS GPS operations than any other country in the world except Thailand. Iran is exceptional with regard to exempting transsexuals from the death penalty if they have had TS GPS (see Section 4.5).

2.7 PUBLIC ACCOMMODATIONS

Transsexual and transgender individuals are sometimes included as part of the GLBT group of people for political advocacy. However, because of their appearance, many transsexual and transgender people cannot hide in plain sight as most GLB can. Many cannot "pass" in public and so are subject to public rejection and harassment because they look different from cultural expectations. With regard to public accommodation, more than 53% of transsexual and transgender individuals report being harassed or disrespected in hotels, airports, and restaurants (Grant et al., 2011). They also report harassment from those government and nongovernment entities that are supposed to assist them. They report denial of equal treatment by government officials at a 22% rate, harassment and disrespect by police at a 29% rate, and denial of equal treatment by court officials at a 12% rate (Grant et al., 2011). Discrimination in public accommodations also applies to public shelters for the homeless and victims of domestic violence. There are a few states and localities that offer protection for transsexuals and transgender people in public accommodations, but it is far from universal.

2.8 LEGAL IDENTIFICATION

Getting appropriate identification documents is a particular problem for transsexuals and transgender people. In the United States, regulations that govern personal identification are not uniform but depend on a patchwork of law, precedent, and local custom. The two main issues for transsexuals are name and gender marker change. Name changes must be granted by state judges in the United States. They are usually routinely granted unless fraud is involved. However, some judges have balked at transsexual name changes because of prejudice, claiming that the person has chosen a name that is inappropriate for his or her sex and therefore fraudulent. Such judges have generally been overruled on appeal, but the added expense and time for transsexuals is burdensome.

In the United States, individual states validate local birth certificates and reissue them if requested. Some states will issue a new birth certificate to transsexuals, but others will issue only an amended birth certificate. Tennessee will not change or amend birth certificate gender markers at all. Amended or uncorrected birth certificates cause future problems in getting other forms of identification and may lead to job discrimination. States also vary with regard to the criteria for name and gender marker change. Some states require confirmation of TS GPS, some states require medical confirmation that the transsexual intends to live exclusively in the new gender role, and some states flatly refuse to change gender markers. Of those transsexuals who complete transition, only 21% are able to complete name and gender marker changes (Grant et al., 2010). Only 59% have been able to change gender markers on state-issued driver's licenses. This means that 41% may not have adequate identification for driving and voting.

The most common form of identification in use in the United States is the driver's license or other state-issued identification. The RealID law is a U.S. federal law that provides requirements for issuance of state licenses. This essentially makes state licenses into national identification cards. They are also valid for identification for air travel, entry to public buildings, and voting. Several pieces of identification can be required to prove name and gender marker, including passports, previous licenses, birth certificates, voter identification cards, and utility bills. State-issued photo identification can be a barrier for transsexual and transgender people to exercise their right to vote. In the 10 states that added additional requirements for photo identification to vote in the 2012 presidential election, it is estimated that more than 27% of transsexuals and transgender people became ineligible to vote in those states (Herman, 2012).

Recently, progress has been made in U.S. passport, Social Security, and veterans identification for gender markers. Passports now only require medical confirmation of the intent to live exclusively in a new gender role at the start of transsexual transition. Social security and the VA will now change the gender marker in their records if requested. For a time, Social Security sent out "no-match" letters to employers if the employer-reported gender marker did not match the employee's gender marker in the Social Security database. This practice resulted in many transsexual and transgender individuals being questioned about their gender. Due to advocacy by the TSTG community, this procedure has been discontinued.

In Europe, many countries still require hormone therapy, TS GPS, sterilization, divorce, and psychiatric testing before transsexuals can change their gender markers on their identification cards (Amnesty International, 2014).

Obtaining appropriate identification papers continues to be a problem for transsexuals and transgender people because of the patchwork of state and agency regulations and the lack of understanding by government officials.

2.9 INCARCERATION

There is no known connection or correlation between TSTG and other behaviors, including criminal behavior. Transsexuals and transgender people are subject to the same biological, environmental, and learning factors that cause people to commit crimes as non-TSTG people. Conversely TSTG are not automatically criminals, although those who engage in street economies are highly visible. Because of family rejection many TSTG are forced into street crime because of their homelessness. However, incarceration of transsexuals and transgender people triggers all kinds of social and political issues because responsibility for the welfare of these prisoners then falls on state and federal governments. Many government officials responsible for the welfare of prisoners have betrayed a notable lack of understanding of TSTG science. Politicians have capitalized on these issues to score points on sociopolitical issues. Transsexual and transgender incarceration reopens the discussion as to whether imprisonment is intended as a punishment or whether it protects society from future crimes. This debate has been carried on for centuries and is still unresolved.

Transsexual and transgender people who are incarcerated for various crimes face physical assault, particularly if assigned to a sex-segregated facility that is inappropriate for their congruent gender behavior predisposition. Physical and sexual assault in jail or prison is a definite problem. In a survey of those transsexual and transgender individuals who had been incarcerated (Grant et al., 2010), 16% of respondents who had been to jail or prison reported being physically assaulted, and 15% reported being sexually assaulted. The authors of this study point to a comparable study that found a sexual assault rate for the general prison population of 4.4% (Jenness, Maxson, Matsuda, & Sumner, 2007). African American respondents reported much higher rates of physical and sexual assault in prison, by both other inmates and corrections officers. Many TSTG individuals are assigned to solitary confinement that has been condemned as injurious to the mental health of prisoners.

Health care for transsexuals in U.S. prisons is a contentious issue, with 17% of those who have been in jail experiencing denial of hormones and 12% experiencing denial of routine health care (Grant et al., 2010). Several lawsuits have been filed to petition for hormones and surgeries during the past few years. Most of them are still in litigation. Thus, transsexual and transgender people who become incarcerated face physical danger and denial of needed health care.

2.10 MILITARY SERVICE

Most countries, including the United States, forbid transsexuals or transgender people from joining their military services. However, many U.S. military members have served without incident with transsexual and transgender soldiers from various NATO countries, including Canada, the United Kingdom, and the Netherlands.

There are undoubtedly many transsexual and transgender people in the U.S. military who work and live in secrecy. As described in Section 2.1, secrecy has human and cultural costs. Transsexual and transgender military soldiers and marines are subject to dismissal and loss of security clearances if they reveal their secret lives. Some seek out help from medical professionals outside the service, which makes them vulnerable to blackmail and dismissal.

In the wake of the repeal of the Don't Ask, Don't Tell law for homosexuality, there is currently impetus to allow transsexual and transgender people to serve openly. This would not require a change in U.S. law, only a change in the armed forces' medical policy. As to whether there is any reason to prevent this from happening, the Palm Center commissioned a national task force study of prominent medical professionals lead by a former U.S. Surgeon General that concluded:

> We find that there is no compelling medical rationale for banning transgender military service, and that eliminating the ban would advance a number of military interests, including enabling commanders to better care for their service members. . . .
>
> Research shows that depriving transgender service members of medically necessary health care poses significant obstacles to their well-being. According to one recent study, "Mental health, medical and substance abuse services obtained outside of the military are supposed to be communicated back to the military, so transgender people who seek these services elsewhere still risk exposure. . . . This leads individuals to go without treatment, allowing symptoms to exacerbate, and causing some to treat symptoms with alcohol or drugs, which could lead to substance abuse or dependence." Research has confirmed, as well, that policies that force individuals to conceal their identities can have significant mental health consequences. (Elders, Steinman, Brown, Coleman, & Kolditz, 2014)

The human cost for transsexual and transgender people is not being able to serve their countries. The cost to military forces is that they lose potential well-motivated volunteers for their workforce. This is demonstrated by the high rate of military enlistment and officership by transsexual and transgender people.

2.11 UNDERSTANDING TSTG SCIENCE

In general, transsexuals and transgender people do not have a good understanding of the science that pertains to them. This leaves them unable to explain or defend their behavior. This is in part a reflection of the inadequacy of science teaching in the United States and other countries, as well as cultural isolation of science from the social sciences, humanities, and the public.

Transsexuals and transgender people need to have an understanding of the TSTG phenomenon to give themselves peace of mind and to know how to educate their medical health professionals about it. Some have taken it upon themselves to try to obtain scientific and medical knowledge to help understand what they are experiencing. Many of these transsexual and transgender individuals are medical doctors and others who would completely understand the science, if it were readily available. One of the aims of this book is to improve the availability of this information.

Many transsexual and transgender advocates and intellectuals seem to adhere to a general cultural resistance about understanding science or educating the public about it, as if science was unknowable. When journalists ask what is the cause of TSTG behavior, these leaders mumble something about it being biological and may cite one of the refuted theories they have read about in the popular press. This leaves them open to criticism by politicians, pseudoscientists, and hate mongers who profit by sensationalizing TSTG issues. Even more important, people in the public sphere end up having useless discussions because the debates are not grounded in scientific definitions or facts.

Many advocates simply use the argument in public appearances that transsexuals and transgender individuals, like all people, deserve their rights. This is true. However, they could also use these appearances to teach some science to the public and dispel the confusion created by the pseudoscientist attacks. In part, the advocates are not to blame because, before this book, there was no comprehensive scientific record of TSTG for them to arm themselves.

Understanding the phenomena of TSTG provides new insights into the human condition. It allows us all to appreciate what it must be like to be another person and reach across the void between people. Understanding TSTG science leads to a celebration of diversity and the insights that TSTG have to offer.

2.12 SUMMARY

Even if one disregards the ethical argument that transsexuals and transgender people should not suffer cultural rejection, the economic costs to a society of such discrimination are considerable. Although there is no overall tally of such costs, several factors can be identified. Ignorance and isolation of science prevent TSTG from fully understanding the phenomenon that they experience and prevent them from using science to defend themselves and obtain their rights. The next chapter begins the presentation of current science regarding TSTG by defining terms and by quantifying the population frequencies of TSTG.

REFERENCES

American College of Obstetricians and Gynecologists. (2011). Healthcare for transgender individuals (Committee Opinion No. 512). *Obstetrics and Gynecology, 118,* 1454–1458.

Amnesty International. (2014). *The state decides who I am*. London: Amnesty International. Retrieved February 7, 2014, from http://www.amnesty.org/en/library/asset/EUR01/001/2014/en/13af83a1-85f5-476f-9fe9-b931f2b2a9f3/eur010012014en.pdf.

Bagby, D. (2013, March 26). Atlanta largest homeless shelter grapples with transgender inclusion. *The Southern Voice*. Retrieved January 1, 2014, from http://womensnet.org.za/news/atlantas-largest-homeless-shelter-grapples-with-transgender-inclusion.html.

Baral, S., Poteat, T., Strömdahl, S., Wirtz, A. L., Guadamuz, T. E., & Beyrer, C. (2013, March). Worldwide burden of HIV in transgender women: A systematic review and meta-analysis. *The Lancet: Infectious Diseases, 13,* 214–222.

Bauer, G., Pyne, J., Fancion, M., & Hammond, R. (2013). Suicidality among trans people in Ontario: Implications for social work and social justice. *Service Social, 59,* 35–62.

Bockting, W., Robinson, B., & Rosser, B. (1998). Transgender HIV prevention: A qualitative needs assessment. *Aids Care, 10,* 505–525.

Boles, J., & Elifson, K. (1994). The social organization of transvestite prostitution and AIDS. *Social Science Medicine, 39,* 85–93.

Clements-Nolle, K., Marx, R., Guzman, R., & Katz, M. (1991, June). HIV prevalence, risk behaviors, health care use and mental health status of transgender persons: Implications for public health intervention. *American Journal of Public Health, 91,* 915–921.

Clements-Nolle, K., Marx, R., & Katz, M. (2006). Attempted suicide among transgender persons: The influence of gender-based discrimination and victimization. *Homosexuality, 51,* 53–59.

Clements-Nolle, K., Wilkinson, W., & Kitanto, M. (2001). HIV prevention and health service needs of the transgender community in San Francisco. In Bockting, W., & Kirk, S. (Eds.), *Transgender and HIV: Risks, prevention and care*. Binghamton, NY: Haworth Press.

Durso, L., & Gates, G. (2012). Serving our youth: Findings from a National Survey of Service Providers working with lesbian, gay, bisexual, and transgender youth who are homeless or at risk of becoming homeless. Los Angeles: The Williams Institute with True Colors Fund and the Palette Fund.

Elders, J., Steinman, A., Brown, G., Coleman, E., & Kolditz, T. (2014, March). *Report of the Transgender Military Service Commission.* San Francisco: The Palm Center.

Gardner, I., & Safer, J. (2013, December). Progress on the road to better medical care for transgender patients. *Current Opinion in Endocrinology, Diabetes & Obesity, 20,* 553–558.

Gay and Lesbian Medical Association. (2014). Guidelines for care of GLBT Patients. Retrieved February 18, 2014, http://www.glma.org/_data/n_0001 /resources/live/Welcoming%20Environment.pdf.

Grant, J., Mottet, L., Tanis, J., Herman, J., Harrison, J., & Keisling, M. (2010, October). *National Transgender Discrimination Survey Report on health and health care. Findings of a Study by the National Center for Transgender Equality and the National Gay and Lesbian Task Force.* Washington, DC: National Center for Transgender Equality and National Gay and Lesbian Task Force.

Grant, J., Mottet, L. A., Tanis, J., with Harrison, J., Herman, J. L., & Keisling, M. (2011). *Injustice at every turn: A report of the National Discrimination Survey.* Washington, DC: National Center for Transgender Equality and National Gay and Lesbian Task Force.

Herman, J. (2012). *The potential impact of voter identification laws on trans-gender voters.* Los Angles: The Williams Institute, UCLA School of Law. Retrieved February 18, 2014, from http://williamsinstitute.law.ucla.edu /wp-content/uploads/Herman-Voter-ID-Apr-2012.pdf.

Herman, J. (2013, September). *Costs and benefits of providing transition-related health care coverage in employee health benefit plans.* Los Angeles: The Williams Institute, UCLA School of Law.

Jenness, V., Maxson, C. L., Matsuda, K. N., & Sumner, J. M. (2007). *Violence in California correctional facilities: An empirical exami-nation of sexual assault.* Irvine, CA: Center for Evidence-Based Cor-rections, Department of Criminology, Law and Society, University of California, Irvine. Retrieved from http://ucicorrections.seweb.uci.edu/pdf /PREA_Presentation_PREA_Report_UCI_Jenness_et_al.pdf.

Kelly, A. (2002). *The psychology of secrets.* New York: Plenum.

Kennedy, N. (2008). Transgendered [*sic*] children in schools: A critical review of homophobic bullying: Safe to learn—embedding anti-bullying work in schools. *Forum, 50,* 383–396.

Kennedy, N., & Helen, M. (2010). Transgender children: More than a theoreti-cal challenge. *Graduate Journal of Social Science, 7,* 26–43.

Kosciw, J., Greytak, E. A., Bartkiewicz, M. J., Boesen, M. J., & Palmer, N. A. (2012). *The 2011 National School Climate Survey.* New York: Gay, Lesbian & Straight Education Network.

Leichtentritt, R. D., & Arad, B. D. (2004). Adolescent and young adult male-to-female transsexuals: Pathways to prostitution. *British Journal of Social Work, 34,* 349–374.

Liu, R., & Mustanski, B. (2001, March). Suicidal ideation and self-harm in lesbian, gay, bisexual, and transgender youth. *American Journal of Preventative Medicine, 42,* 221–228.

Make the Road. (2010, March). Transgender need not apply: A report on gender identity job discrimination. *Make the Road,* 1–22. Retrieved from http://www.maketheroad.org/pix_reports/TransNeedNotApplyReport_05.10.pdf.

Mustanski, B., & Liu, R. (2010, April). A longitudinal study of predictors of suicide attempt among lesbian, gay, bisexual and transgender youth. *Archives of Sexual Behavior, 42,* 437–448.

Mustanski, B., & Liu, R. (2013). A longitudinal study of predictors of suicide attempts among lesbian, gay, bisexual and transgender youth. *Archives of Sexual Behavior, 42,* 437–448.

Nuttbrook, L., Rosenblum, A., & Blumentstein, R. (2002). *International Journal of Transgenderism, 6*(4). Retrieved February 2014 from http://www.iiav.nl/ezines/web/ijt/97-03/numbers/symposion/ijtvo06no04_03.htm.

Obedin-Maliver, J., Goldsmith, E. S., Stewart, L., White, W., Tran, E., Brenman, S., et al. (2011). Lesbian, gay, bisexual and transgender-related content in undergraduate medical education. *JAMA, 306,* 971–977.

Pang, H., Pugh, K., & Catalan, J. (1994). Gender identity disorder and HIV disease. *International Journal of the Study of STD and AIDS, 5,* 130–132.

Quintana, N., Rosenthal, J., & Krehely, J. (2010, June). *On the streets: The federal response to gay and transgender homeless youth.* Center for American Progress. Retrieved February 6, 2014, from http://www.americanprogress.org/wp-content/uploads/issues/2010/06/pdf/lgbtyouthhomelessness.pdf.

Rotondi, N. K., Bauer, G. R., Travers, R., Travers, A., Scanlon, K., & Kaay, M. (2011). Depression in male-to-female transgender Ontarians. *Canadian Journal of Community Mental Health, 30,* 113–133.

Sausa, L. A., Keatley, J. A., & Operario, D. (2007). Perceived risks and benefits of sex work among transgender women of color in San Francisco. *Archives of Sexual Behavior, 36,* 768–777.

Schepel, E. (2011). *A comparative study of adult transgender and female prostitution.* Arizona State University. Retrieved February 6, 2014, from http://repository.asu.edu/attachments/56451/content/Schepel_asu_0010N_10422.pdf.

Spicer, S. (2010). Healthcare needs of the transgender homeless population. *Journal of Gay and Lesbian Health, 14,* 320–339.

Studwell, K. (2013, January). NIH continues implementation of IOM's recommendations for LGBTI health research. *Psychological Science Agenda*. Retrieved July 7, 2014, from http://www.apa.org/science/about/psa/2013/01/lgbti-research.aspx.

Testa, R., Sciacca, L. M., Wang, F., Hendricks, M. L., Goldblum, P., Bradford, J., & Bongar, B. (2012, August). Effects of violence on transgender people. *Professional Psychology: Research and Practice, 4,* 452–459.

Transgender Law and Policy Institute. (2014). Non-discrimination laws that include gender identity and expression. Retrieved February 18, 2014, from http://transgenderlaw.org/ndlaws/index.htm#jurisdictions.

Veterans Health Administration, Department of Veterans Affairs. (2011, June 9). *Providing health care for transgender and intersex veterans* (VHA Directive 2011-024). Retrieved April 29, 2014, from http://www.va.gov/vhapublications/ViewPublication.asp?pub_ID=2863.

Wood, A., Linley, P. A., Maltby, J., Baliousis, M., & Joseph, S. (2008). The authentic personality: A theoretical and empirical conceptualization and the development of the authenticity scale. *Journal of Counseling Psychology, 55,* 385–399.

Wright, J. (2008, December 26). Trans woman's death shines light on plight of homeless. *The Dallas Voice.*

3

Definitions and Population Frequencies

3.0 INTRODUCTION

Before we examine the evidence from various scientific disciplines to help understand transsexualism and transgenderism (TSTG), there are two important topics that need to be covered. The first deals with defining biopsychology terms that can be used in standardizing science across multiple scientific disciplines; the second involves understanding population frequencies for TSTG to help interpret scientific results. The results of these two topics provide scientific tools that will be helpful in understanding TSTG in subsequent chapters.

Because terminology often varies widely between investigators and in the general public, it is important to define some important terms to maintain scientific consistency. TSTG is defined as a phenomenon in which the gender behavior or verbal declaration of gender identity of an individual is incongruent with their assigned natal gender behavior category and congruent with some other gender behavior category. To fully understand this definition, it is necessary to provide additional definitions and explanations. A common barrier to understanding this definition is that there is confusion and conflation between the terms *sex* and *gender*. This conflation leads to scientific ambiguity.

The second topic of interest concerns population frequencies for transsexuals and transgender people. Such frequencies are often used to interpret scientific results in the literature. Errors in interpretation can be made if these frequencies are not accurate. Until 2000, all of the estimates of population frequency were based on clinical observations that vastly underestimated the frequency of TSTG. Most transsexual and transgender individuals were never counted in these clinical observations because they felt no need to see a mental health professional. Better estimates of TSTG population frequencies were made using engineering mathematical estimation theory in 2000. For the first time, population frequencies were accurately estimated using a scientific method. The results of these engineering studies indicated that TSTG occurs much more frequently than older estimates would suggest. Subsequent population surveys have supported these engineering estimates.

3.1 DEFINITIONS

3.1.1 Transsexualism and Transgenderism

Transsexualism and Transgenderism is a phenomenon in which the gender behavior or verbal declaration of gender identity of an individual is incongruent with their assigned natal gender behavior category and congruent with some other gender behavior category. Gender behavior category is typically determined by natal sex, but some cultures also use gender identity.

To understand this definition, it is necessary to define and discuss several supporting terms (these supporting terms are defined in subsequent sections):

- Gender and sex
- Gender versus sex
- Gender identity
- Gender behavior categories
- Transsexualism and transgenderism

3.1.1.1 Gender and Sex

Gender refers to behavior, not to sex organs. To differentiate behavior from sex, the term gender was borrowed from language grammars in which each noun is typically assigned to masculine, feminine, or neuter category declensions. **Gender behavior** refers to behaviors that are associated with culturally defined **gender behavior categories**. In contemporary binary gender systems, the feminine gender behavior category refers to girl/woman/she and the masculine gender refers to boy/man/he. For example, the gender behavior of men usually includes having short hair, whereas women and girls have longer hairstyles. Women often wear lipstick and nail polish, and men do not. We can regard gender behaviors as tasks that culture expects people to perform in accordance with their assigned gender behavior category. The rules and behaviors in gender behavior categories are somewhat arbitrary and vary from culture to culture and time to time. There are also **nonbinary gender systems** with multiple gender behavior categories. Gender and sex are not equivalent. In fact, the term gender was borrowed specifically to differentiate gender behavior from sex.

The scientific use of the term **sex** originates in biology, and its meaning and uses are well understood in that discipline. In the TSTG biopsychology context, sex refers to **sex organs**, including **primary sex organs** such as genitalia and **secondary sex organs** such as the brain and nervous system. These are the organs involved in sexual arousal, sexual behavior, and intercourse that can result in human reproduction, although humans have sex for reasons other than reproduction. Assignment to a single sex category based on inspection of primary sex organs is typically required by culture and societies, but assignment at birth to these categories is not always straightforward (see Section 3.1.4). The **biological sex categories** are **male** and female. In biology, male and female are defined by the size of their gametes, which are the cells that fuse together in conception. Males usually have smaller gametes than females. Secondary sex organs have functions other than sexual intercourse but are nonetheless important for an understanding of TSTG. They include the brain and nervous system as well as the five senses.

Sexual behavior includes behavior that potentially can lead to intercourse as well as intercourse itself. Some gender behaviors may serve to trigger sexual arousal and behavior. The definition of sex used in this book is compatible with biological definitions.

3.1.1.2 Sex versus Gender

Repurposing the word gender to differentiate it from sex has had several positive effects. For TSTG, it meant that old cultural stereotypes such as the required yoking of sex assignment to gender behavior categories, so-called **cisgenderism,** could be violated. Transsexuals and transgender people could have male bodies but practice feminine behavior or female bodies and practice masculine behavior. For science, it meant that gender behavior could be studied separately from sex and sexual behavior, providing increased precision. For feminists, it allowed them to assert that gender behavior was separate from sex and that it was culturally constructed. The term *gender* is a valuable tool and should not be conflated with sex.

One of the barriers to understanding TSTG is the confusion between the terms *sex* and *gender* because the definition of TSTG involves both concepts. Sex and gender are not the same. The definitions of **sex** and **gender** have become increasingly conflated in the past two decades, robbing them of the scientific precision (Pearson, 1996) necessary to help understand TSTG and other phenomena. Strangely, the conflation began with social science researchers, who should have known better given the care with which behavioral terms are usually defined. The conflation now extends beyond social science into the public media. Gender is essentially used as a polite term for sex, as if to deny that sex exists. Transsexuals and transgender people know about this confusion and, in explaining TSTG, they often refer to the phrase "sex is between the legs and gender is between the ears." That is not quite precise enough for use in science, but the ideas in the phrase are headed in the right direction. To reiterate, the term *sex* concerns sex organs, and the term *gender* concerns behavior.

3.1.1.3 Gender Identity

The term **gender identity** was coined by Stoller (1964) and involves verbal declarations of feelings of congruence with a particular gender behavior category. Gender identity is an expression of which gender behavior category a person believes they[1] should belong. Current Western cultures assign gender behavior categories at birth based on sex assignment at birth, but other cultures make this assignment during childhood based on behavior and verbalized gender identity.

3.1.1.4 Gender Behavior Categories

Gender behavior categories are sets of gender behaviors that are explicitly or implicitly determined by culture to organize, categorize, and stereotype people. Gender behavior categories involve behavioral tasks, roles, rules, and norms. People are expected to adhere to their culturally assigned category by culture, and some rules are typically codified by governments. Most Western cultures have two gender behavior categories, but some historical cultures had three or four, and one current culture has five (see Chapter 4). Some historic North American Native American cultures allowed certain of their members to move back and forth between gender behavior categories and are generally termed "**two-spirit**." These people were revered for their wisdom and were frequently skilled in the tasks involved in more than one gender behavior category. One day they would have a feminine presentation and

---

[1] Note that in this book for scientific precision, I sometimes use the neutral *they* and *their* pronouns as the singular because the book content concerns both binary and nonbinary gender systems. Nonbinary gender systems sometimes have as many as three, four, or even five gender behavior categories. For this reason, it would be misleading and scientifically incorrect to use singular pronouns from the Western binary gender system. English gender-neutral singular pronoun systems have been suggested, but none of them have reached acceptance.

weave cloth, the next day they wore masculine clothing to engage in warfare. Their wisdom is attributed to experiencing both gender behavior categories and learning about people in each category. Because of this wisdom, two-spirits often occupied roles of medicine man or shaman. We describe cultures with multiple behavior categories and two-spirits in Chapter 4. Gender behavior categories are constructed by cultures, not by biology, and gender systems vary between cultures.

The tasks, rules, and norms of behavior categories vary from culture to culture both historically and geographically. They are somewhat arbitrary in many cases. Historically, male soldiers in the English Cavalier era were expected to have long hair, but this norm changed when Cromwell expected his soldiers to have short hair, the so-called Roundheads. In modern times, this has been taken to the extreme by requiring crew cuts for male soldiers. Violation of gender behavior category rules is sometimes done for effect. An example is the long hair and exaggerated, sometimes feminine, makeup of male rock musicians.

A classic example of the arbitrary nature of gender behavior category rules is using pink clothing for girls and blue clothing for boys. Before World War I, children mostly wore white because it was interchangeable between children. If anything there was a tendency for girls to wear blue and boys to wear pink. Sometime between World War I and World War II the rule of pink for girls caught on, encouraged by manufacturers who wanted to sell more children's clothing (Paoletti, 2012). By World War II, the Nazis were already using pink badges to identify homosexuals because of the (inaccurate) stereotype that all homosexuals display feminine behavior. Despite a few years of feminist rebellion in the 1960s, the convention has continued to grow (Waterlow, 2013).

We consider gender behavior categories in more detail in Chapters 4, 8, and 10. Most people find it surprising that children learn the basics of gender behavior categories by age 2 years. Learning gender behavior categories is a prerequisite for TSTG. The learning continues into early adulthood. Culturally defined gender behavior categories are arbitrary and vary from time to time and culture to culture.

3.1.1.5 Transsexualism and Transgenderism

The terms *transsexual* and *transgender* only came into common usage in the 1960s. Before that time, several other terms were used to define, sometimes incorrectly, the TSTG phenomenon. Some are still in use today, so it is necessary to distinguish them from the terms transsexualism and transgenderism.

Terminology for TSTG has evolved over the past century to reflect the incorrect belief that those who violated gender behavior categories did so for sexual arousal and gratification. Magnus Hershfeld, an early 20th-century

German sexologist coined the term **transvestite** based on the Latin for "cross-dress": *trans*, the preposition for "across," and *vestita*, "clothed." In German, this coined term would not have a sexual connotation, but Hershfeld immediately created a connotation for this word by defining it as dressing for sexual arousal and pleasure. Both Hershfeld and clinicians who followed in his school believed that sexual arousal was the cause of TSTG. It was naturally included in the list of sexual fetishes when the concept of fetish came into vogue in the 1940s. A **sexual fetish** involves sexual arousal from exposure to inanimate objects. We now know that sexual arousal sometimes accompanies TSTG when opposite-gender clothing is worn, but it is not a fetish and not a causal factor in TSTG, as described in Chapters 9 and 12. Today, *transvestite* is regarded as a pejorative word and is used primarily in degradation of transsexuals and transgender people.

The term *transvestite* was largely replaced in the mid-20th century by the word **cross-dresser**. Unlike transvestite, the term *cross-dresser* does not assume a sexual fetish or sexual arousal. Today, cross-dresser refers to a wide range of behaviors, not just TSTG behavior. It can be used to refer to **drag queens** and **drag kings** who cross-dress for theatrical performances, cross-dressing for political protest, and cross-dressing by male models to promote feminine clothing and makeup. There are also female models who cross-dress to promote masculine clothing.

Drag queens and drag kings generally cross-dress for entertainment purposes, but if an individual maintains cross-dressing behavior in nonperforming situations or expresses transsexual or transgender gender identity, they should be considered transsexual or transgender. Drag is about the performance, and although most drag queens are male homosexuals, many are male heterosexuals; a few are natal females as well.

The term **transsexual** was introduced by Cauldwell (1949) and popularized by Harry Benjamin (1966) who first outlined professional standards for transsexual transition. The term **transgender** was coined by John Oliven (1965) and was popularized by various transgender people who pioneered the concept and practice of transgenderism. It is sometimes said that Virginia Prince (1976) popularized the term, but history shows that many transgender people advocated use of this term much more than Prince. The adjective *transgendered* should not be used because transsexuals and transgender people regard it as an indication of victimization.

Transsexuals constitute a subset of transgender people. To date, there is insufficient science to differentiate between transsexualism and transgenderism. The behavior is the same, but the frequency, duration, and degree of voluntary body change differs. Some transgender people only occasionally engage in behavior that is incongruent with their natal assigned gender behavior category, whereas transsexuals usually engage in it on a nearly continuous basis. Using the behavioral definition of overt behavior is scientifically conservative because it does not rely on intervening variables that cannot be measured.

The term **tranny** is a pejorative term that originated by contraction in the 1970s. It is beginning to be reclaimed by transsexual and transgender people just as the pejorative *queer* has been reclaimed by people who are **gender-queer** (discussed later). It is acceptable to use *tranny* only if you are a transsexual or transgender, and even then some may take offense.

Transsexuals and transgender males are known as **male-to-female** (MTF) or **transwomen**, and transsexual and transgender females are known as **female-to-male** (FTM) or **transmen**. Transsexuals and transgender people prefer to be addressed with the pronouns that are consistent with their preferred gender behavior category. For example FTM strongly prefer masculine pronouns, and MTF strongly prefer feminine pronouns. If a person's gender behavior category is not obvious, it is polite to ask transsexual and transgender people which pronouns they prefer. Professional rules for journalists have attempted to enforce this pronoun etiquette, although many publications and blogs ignore it. Some unethical journalists deliberately use the wrong pronouns to degrade transsexuals and transgender people for sensationalism. Transsexuals and transgender people prefer terms that are associated with their congruent gender behavior category.

Gender identity disorder was a pathological clinical term indicating that TSTG behavior itself was a disorder. It has been replaced by **gender dysphoria** in the current list of clinical terms used for diagnosis known as the *Diagnostic and Statistical Manual of Mental Disorders*. Gender dysphoria simply means that a person is not happy with their assigned gender behavior category (dysphoria is the opposite of euphoria in Greek). It is regarded as less pathological, but TSTG remains on the list in other forms, unlike homosexuality, for example, which was deleted in 1974 (see Section 12.2).

Although the definition of TSTG provided earlier largely relies on observable behavior, the capability to directly measure internal physiological TSTG phenomena should improve with future instrumentation as neuroscience progresses. As an example, we are already starting to see functional magnetic resonance imaging (fMRI) studies that compare TSTG brain response with non-TSTG brain response for such things as reaction to visual erotic stimuli (Gizewski, Krause, Wanke, Forsting, & Senf, 2006; Gizewski et al., 2009), mental rotation tasks (Schöning et al., 2010), spatial cognition (Schöning et al., 2010), and emotional patterns (Ku et al., 2013; see Chapter 10, this volume). Although all of the brain processes involved with TSTG and gender identity are not currently observable, they may become so in the future.

As a result of the information in this section, a definition of TSTG emerges that describes the interactions between biological bases for TSTG and cultural gender behavior categories.

3.1.2 Gender Predisposition

There is evidence to support the idea that TSTG behavior results from an incongruence between **gender predisposition** and assigned gender behavior category. Humans are known to have all sorts of predispositions, for example, the capability to learn language, right- or left-handedness, musical ability, intelligence, overall physical activity level, sexual orientation, and susceptibility to particular diseases. Gender predisposition means that one has biological tendencies to perform certain gender behaviors and not others. When the behaviors resulting from gender behavior predisposition and the assigned gender behavior category are incongruent and in conflict, TSTG may result. For it to be classified as TSTG, the individual must find and follow a congruent gender behavior category. Those who do not find a congruent gender behavior category sometimes identify as **genderqueer**. Most cultures have a binary **gender system** in which there are only two gender behavior categories. Males are supposed to behave according to the masculine gender behavior category, and females are supposed to behave according to the feminine gender behavior category. This orthodoxy is termed **cisgender**. Some cultures have several gender behavior categories that provide more alternatives to children and adults. Some cultures allow people to move freely from one gender behavior category to another depending on the individual and the demands of the society. An example is the North American Native "two-spirit" tradition noted earlier.

The evidence to establish **biological gender predisposition** is detailed in later chapters, but a summary follows. First, diverse biological gender predispositions are ubiquitous among cultures both historically and geographically, as described in Chapter 4, indicating a biological gender predisposition. Second, there is good scientific evidence that indicates that the primary causal factors for TSTG are DNA genetics (Chapter 5) and possible epigenetics (Chapter 6) that are at work from conception onward. Third, knowledge of TSTG emerges when a child is 3 or 4 years old, leaving little time for factors other than genetics and epigenetics to be at work. Fourth, the only other possible causal factor for TSTG based on its early realization is early parental child rearing, but there is ample evidence to reject this, as presented in Chapter 8. Fifth, "natural experiments" happened in which children are reared in the opposite gender from their birth sex due to intersex or accidental conditions but indicate discomfort with their assigned gender (Colapinto, 2006; Diamond & Beh, 2008; Reiner & Gearhart, 2004). In the famous case of David Reimer, the parents attempted to raise a male child as a girl after a circumcision accident and genital surgery. The result was rejection of his assigned gender behavior predisposition and eventual suicide. Another case in the literature describes a situation similar to that of David Reimer; this individual has a history of "tomboyism" and at one point declared a "bisexual" sexual identity (Bradley,

Oliver, Chernick, & Zucker, 1998). Finally, neuroanatomical and functional brain differences have been found by comparing those with TSTG with non-TSTG in MRI and fMRI experiments (see Chapter 10). The biological basis for TSTG is mediated through the gender predisposition of individuals.

3.1.3 Sexual Arousal

Sexual arousal involves physiological preparation of the sex organs for sexual behavior. Examples of preparatory responses are penile erection and vaginal secretion. Sexual arousal is stimulated by particular stimuli and is learned through classical conditioning. Classical or Pavlovian conditioning involves repeated pairing of a stimulus with sexual arousal. How sexual arousal is learned is described in detail in Chapter 9. Understanding sexual arousal is important for an understanding of TSTG because many people mistakenly believe that transsexuals and transgender people cross-dress to become sexually aroused. However, stimuli lose their ability to evoke sexual arousal with repeated exposure, yet TSTG persist in their behavior. Interviews with transsexuals and transgender people indicate that sexual arousal is not a primary reason for cross-dressing (Buhrich, 1978).

3.1.4 Intersex, or Differences in Sexual Development

An understanding of TSTG science requires references to science concerning **intersex** conditions or **differences in sexual development (DSD)**. A surprisingly large number of babies are born with these differences, which sometimes result in indeterminate natal sex. Depending on the phenomena one includes in the intersex population, intersex population frequencies vary between .05%, .66%, and 1.9% of live births, but some estimates are as high as 4% (Costello, 2012; Morgan, 2012). DSDs are mostly due to genetic and epigenetic causal factors, some of which are well understood from medical research.

Some of these anomalies result in over- or undersecretion of testosterone, which some investigators hypothesize to be potential causal factors in TSTG. We examine such claims in Chapter 6.

Note that some subcultures and countries prefer the term *intersex*, whereas others prefer *DSD*, so it is polite to ask which should be used. People with these differences strongly reject the old term *disorders of sexual development* because these differences are seen as naturally occurring and not pathological.

3.1.5 Sexual Orientation

Sexual orientation refers to attraction and sexual arousal by a person to the same or opposite sex for the purposes of sexual behavior. The current acceptable terms are **gay** and **lesbian**, although gay is increasingly being used to refer to lesbians as well. People who are **bisexual** are attracted to both sexes. The causal factors that determine sexual orientation to one or the other sex are suspected and some of the available evidence is summarized in Section 12.1.3.4.

TSTG may be attracted to the same or opposite sex (Blanchard, 1989; Chivers & Bailey, 2000), but there is no indication that homosexuality causes TSTG. They appear to be independent phenomena (see Section 12.1.3.4). However, sexual orientation should be taken into account in the design and conduct of scientific studies of TSTG because the causal factors and mechanisms involved with sexual orientation may be confounded with those involved with TSTG. There are examples of this experimental design confound in Section 6.1 that were later resolved. Some transsexuals and transgender people start out as heterosexual and some as homosexual. The difference may help clinicians predict the time course of the emergence of transsexualism because some early homosexuals tend to become transsexual at an earlier age. Some transsexuals change their sexual orientation during transition after hormone therapy or genital plastic surgery, as described in Section 13.4.

3.1.6 Transsexual Transition

Transsexual transition involves semipermanent or permanent voluntary body changes to make sex organs look more male or more female and help bring TSTG presentation into alignment with cultural expectations of the congruent gender behavior category of a transsexual.

Transsexual transition is discussed in detail in Chapter 13. Transsexual transition involves well-defined and disciplined medical procedures. The **World Professional Association for Transgender Health** is the governing body that provides guidelines for health care professionals with regard to transsexual transition and treatment. MTF may take female sex hormones known as **hormone therapy** (HT), reduce body hair through electrolysis, have breast implant surgery, and may have **facial feminization surgery** (FFS) or other procedures. FTM may have their breasts removed, known as **top surgery**, and take male sex hormones (HT). Transsexual transition involves a set of procedures, some of which nontranssexual transgender people also have performed, such as breast augmentation.

Transition culminates in **TS genital plastic surgery** (GPS) although less than 25% to 35% of transsexuals ever get such surgery. TS GPS is even less frequent for FTM because FTM GPS is still being perfected. GPS may be performed in several stages or performed in one operation. Of course, TS GPS is a 20th-century invention. Before GPS, castration was used to create eunuchs for harem administration and to preserve the soprano/contralto voices of males in choirs (known as **castrati**). Although TS GPS is not perfect in changing sex organs, externally it is quite advanced. It is sometimes difficult for even physicians to discern that MTF surgeries have been performed. Medical technologies are increasingly available that someday may be useful for TSTG. Recently, uterine transplants have been performed in natal females (Johannesson, 2014). Uterine transplants between females are expected to produce a live birth sometime in 2014. Artificial vaginas have been successfully grown in the laboratory and implanted into natal females (Raya-Rivera et al., 2014).

TS GPS has been called by various names, but most of them are misnomers. *Sexual reassignment surgery* is a misnomer because the change in sex organs is currently incomplete and primarily cosmetic. *Gender reassignment surgery* and *gender confirmation surgery* are misnomers because the person's congruent gender does not change and the terms confound sex and gender. *Genital reconstruction surgery* is a misnomer because the person's genitals are not restored to a previous configuration. Thus, the most correct and general term is simply TSTG genital plastic surgery. This term applies to anyone, whether transsexual/transgender or not; some nontransgender people have GPS for cosmetic or medical reasons, although the surgery is usually less extensive.

After completion of transsexual transition, some transsexuals change their names, move geographically, and establish new social relations. This is known as living in **stealth**. In the United States, it is becoming increasingly difficult to do this because of security procedures aimed at controlling identity documentation. There are also onerous procedures for changing birth certificates and identity documents in many states due to cultural rejection (see Chapter 2). There is now a trend away from living in stealth. TSTG advocates, who believe that transsexuals need to be visible to obtain TSTG rights, welcome this trend.

3.2 POPULATION FREQUENCIES

Knowledge of TSTG **population frequencies** is important for understanding the phenomenon. Population frequencies indicate that TSTG is too frequent to be ignored in public policies in part because of the economic impacts discussed in Chapter 2. Accurate population frequencies are needed to analyze and interpret scientific findings as discussed in other chapters. In the past, investigators made claims about their findings on TSTG causation based on the mistakenly believed extreme rarity of TSTG. Our knowledge of TSTG population frequencies has become more accurate now that estimation and survey approaches have augmented clinical intake frequencies.

Accurate population frequency data are difficult to achieve from clinical sources because most transsexuals and transgender people are never treated for TSTG by a mental health professional. Furthermore, many transsexuals do not always seek medical permission to transition. Do-it-yourself hormone groups exist that share information on transitioning. With regard to HT, many countries do not require a prescription from a physician to sell hormones. One can also readily buy hormones on the black market. Clinical statistics do not always reflect transsexual GPS done abroad in countries where procedures can be cheaper or more accessible (a practice known as medical tourism). Wait times in the United Kingdom drive transsexuals to travel to Thailand or Morocco. In the early days of recording TSTG statistics, definitions of what constituted a transsexual or transgender person varied from country to country and from investigator to investigator.

Things changed starting in 2001, when a world-class research engineer, familiar with statistical estimation procedures, quickly performed some statistical sanity checks on traditional clinical frequencies. The clinical frequencies were found to grossly understate the frequencies of MTF TSTG (Conway 2001–2002; Kelly, 2001; Olyslager & Conway, 2007). Conway proceeded to conduct formal engineering estimation procedures. Instead of counting patients coming through the clinic door, they estimated population frequencies based on the rate of TS GPS by all doctors offering operations to estimate the rate of transsexualism and the numbers of transgender people attending support group meetings to estimate the rate of transgenderism. They provided the first statistically precise and accurate estimates of lower bounds for MTF TSTG. These lower bounds were still several orders of magnitude higher for both MTF transsexualism and MTF transgenderism compared with previous clinical estimates.

In the past decade, partly because of more enlightened public policy for TSTG, surveys of the population were taken to estimate the future treatment capacities needed for TSTG. Several countries with government-operated health care performed such surveys to ensure that they have the capacity to treat the volume of future transsexuals and transgender people. The engineering estimates served as useful comparisons. Surveys of TSTG have limitations, just like all surveys do, but there are some particular problems with regard to surveying TSTG. For example, some transsexuals and transgender people may not admit their status due to fear of cultural rejection including loss of their jobs and families. Population surveys provide a new source of information as acceptance of TSTG has improved.

3.2.1 MTF Transsexual Population Frequencies

A summary of population frequency studies for MTF transsexualism is shown in Table 3.1. Referencing this table, the studies from 1968 to 2001 were generally clinical studies, primarily based on transsexualism statistics at clinics in non-U.S. countries. The one exception was a passport marker change study that occurred early in the German Transsexual Program. These statistics greatly underestimated the transsexual population as many investigators understood at the time and they so reported. Historically, the population statistics cited publicly are derived from the results of these early clinical studies. As can be seen by inspection, the criteria for inclusion in the study as transsexual varied greatly, from intake to transsexualism diagnosis to hormone administration and TS GPS. But by the mid-1990s some estimates were an order of magnitude higher in frequency than earlier studies.

Conway, Kelly, and Olyslager conducted their engineering mathematical estimation studies from 2001 through 2007, radically changing the scientific information on the rarity of transsexualism. As shown, they carefully calculated the population frequency of TS for various objective criteria. The frequencies jumped two orders of magnitude from historical studies. The study by Horton (2008) had somewhat lower clinical estimates, but they were on the same order of magnitude as the engineer. Subsequent studies have also been clinical or passport marker changes, which are all 1 to 2 orders of magnitude higher than the earliest studies. The studies by Reed were surveys of clinicians across the United Kingdom to assist the National Health Service.

Because of the diversity of the design of these studies, it is impractical to conduct a thorough meta-analysis combining all of the results. However, by inspection, a good rule of thumb for MTF transsexualism is a population frequency of 0.1% or higher. Some values are higher, and some are lower, but that percentage appears to be within the right order of magnitude for the population at large, given the most rigorous and most current findings.

3.2.2 MTF TG Population Frequencies

A summary of population frequency studies for MTF transgenderism is shown in Table 3.2. As we can see from the table, studies for transgenderism had a later historical start than those for transsexualism, probably because the term *transgender* was not introduced until the late 1960s, and it took some time for it to enter common usage and to be understood by clinicians.

From Conway (2001–2002) and Kuyper and Wijsen (2013), it can be judged that the lower bound of transgenderism is at least 1% to 5%. Two studies indicate that approximately 5% of males have tried cross-dressing. Although the clinical studies have lower rates as expected, the Conway (2001–2002) results were two to three orders of magnitude higher. And the Reed study indicates that UK estimates from transgender clubs is in the same order of magnitude as the Conway, Kelly, and Olyslager studies.

Again because of the diversity of the design of these studies, it is impractical to conduct a meta-analysis combining these results. However, we will use a rule of thumb for the purposes of this book for MTF TG as a 1% population frequency. Some values are higher, some lower, but that figure appears to be in the right order of magnitude and, according to Conway (2001–2002), establishes a lower bound.

Table 3.1. Summary of population frequency studies for male-to-female transsexualism. *Note:* Eklund et al. reference is for reports for 1980 and 1986. FTM = female-to-male; GPS = genital plastic surgery; HT = hormone therapy; MTF = male-to-female; postop = postoperative; TS = transsexualism.

Year	Author(s)	Location	TG/TS	Type	MTF/FTM Ratio	Criterion	Odds	Percent
1968	Walinder	Sweden	TS	Clinical Diagnosis	MTF		1:37000	0.003
1968	Pauly	World	TS	Postop	MTF		1:100000	0.001
1974	Hoenig, and Kenna	England/Wales	TS	Clinical diagnosis	MTF		1:34000	0.003
1980	Eklund et al.	Netherlands	TS	HT	MTF		1:45000	0.002
1981	Ross et al.	Australia	TS	Clinical	MTF	Psychiatrist survey	1:24000	0.004
1986	Eklund et al.	Netherlands	TS	HT	MTF		1:18000	0.006
1993	Bakker et al.	Netherlands	TS	Diagnosed TS	MTF		1:11900	0.008
1996	Weitze & Osbur	Germany	TS	Passport change	MTF		1:42000	0.024
1996	van Kesteren et al.	Netherlands	TS	Clinical	MTF		1:11900	0.008
1998	Tsoi	Singapore	TS	Seeking surgery	MTF		1:2900	0.034
1999	Wilson et al.	Scotland	TS	HT	MTF	TS HT	3.33/100000	0.003
1999	Wilson et al.	Scotland	TS	Postop	MTF	TS postop	4.5/100000	0.005
2001	Conway	United States	TS	Postop	MTF	Lower bound	1/2500	0.040
2001	Conway	United States	TS	TS	MTF	Lower bound	1/500	0.200

2001	Conway	TS	TS preoperative	MTF	Lower bound	1:375	0.267
2001	Conway	TS	TS transitioners	MTF	Lower bound	1:170	0.588
2001	Kelly	TS	TS postop	MTF	Lower bound	1:750	0.133
2006	Gómez Gil et al.	TS	Clinical diagnosis	MTF		1:21031	0.005
2007	Zucker et al.	TS	Public survey	MTF	Wishes opposite sex	1:100	1.000
2007	Zucker et al.	TS	Public survey	MTF	Wishes opposite sex	1:29	3.500
2007	DeCupere et al.	TS	Postop	MTF	Lower bound	1:12900	0.008
2007	Olyslager & Conway	TS	TS	MTF	Lower bound	1:200–1:250	0.500
2007	Olyslager & Conway	TS	GPS	MTF	Lower bound	1:2500	0.040
2008	Horton	TS	Clinical postop incidence	MTF	U.S. GPS MD Survey	1:190000	0.001
2008	Horton	TS	Postop	MTF	U.S. GPS MD Survey	1:2500	0.400
2008	Horton	TS	Preop	MTF	U.S. GPS MD Survey	1:750	0.133
2008	Reed et al.	TS	Clinical incidence	MTF		2.6/100000	0.003
2008	Reed et al.	TS	Clinical incidence	MTF		21/100000	0.021
2008	Veale	TS	Passport change	MTF		1:3639	0.027
2009	Reed et al.	TS	Clinical intake	MTF		16/100000	0.016
2010	Brain	TS	Passport change	MTF		1:1500	0.067

Table 3.2. Summary of population frequency studies for male-to-female transgenderism. DSM-IV = *Diagnostic and Statistical Manual of Mental Disorders*, 4th ed.; FTM = female-to-male; GID = gender identity disorder; LGBT = lesbian, gay, bisexual, and transgender; MTF = male-to-female; TS = transsexualism; TG = transgenderism.

Year	Author(s)	Location	TG/TS	Type	MTF/FTM	Criterion/Notes	Odds	Percent
1997	Zucker et al.	Canada	TG	Opposite sex preference	MTF	Children	1:100	1.000
1999	Wilson et al.	Scotland	TG	Clinical intake	MTF	No treatment	3.27/100000	0.003
1999	Wilson et al.	Scotland	TG	Counseling	MTF	GID counseling	2.34/100000	0.002
2001	Conway	United States	TG	TG	MTF	Lower bound	1:20 1:50	5.000
2001	Kelly	UK	TG	TG transitioners	MTF	Lower bound	1:3750	0.027
2001	Reed et al.	Netherlands	TG	Have cross-dressed	MTF		1:100 1:20	1–5
2001	Conway	United States	TG	TS transitioners	MTF	Lower bound	1:200	0.500
2002	Coolidge	United States	TG	Twin study GID DSM-IV ratings	Combined	Recruited by newspaper	2.3/200	2.300
2002	Winter	Hong Kong	TG	Counting Kathoey	MTF	Behavioral observation	6/1000	0.600
2004	Bye et al.	US: California	TG	LGBT tobacco phone survey	Combined	Lower bound	1:50	2.000
2004	Bye et al.	US: California	TG	LGBT tobacco survey	Combined	Lower bound	1:50	2.000
2005	Langstrom & Zucker	Sweden	TG	Clinical	MTF	Survey TG aroused	1:4348	0.023

Year	Author	Country		Description	Type	Note	Ratio	Value
2006	van Beijsterveldt et al.	Netherlands	TG	Twins at 7 years old	MTF	Cross-gender behavior by mothers	1:31	3.200
2006	van Beijsterveldt et al.	Netherlands	TG	Twins at 10 years old	MTF	Cross-gender behavior by mothers	1:40	2.400
2007	Olyslager & Conway	United States	TG	TG	MTF		1:100	1.000
2008	Horton	United States	TG	Clinical GID	MTF		1:1500	0.067
2009	Reed et al.	UK	TG	Estimate from clubs	MTF		1:100	1.000
2011	Gates	United States	TG	Review of surveys	Combined		1:333	0.300
2012	Clark et al.	New Zealand	TG	Youth survey	MTF		1:83	1.200
2012	Conron et al.	US: Massachusetts	TG	Health survey	Combined	Lower bound	1:212	0.467
2013	Shields et al.	United States	TG	Middle school survey	Combined		1:77	1.300
2013	Kuyper & Wijsen	Netherlands	TG	Population survey	MTF	Equal gender identity	1:22	4.600
2013	Kuyper & Wijsen	Netherlands	TG	Population survey	MTF	Stronger with opposite sex	1:91	1.100
2013	Shields et al.	US: California	TG	Middle school survey	Combined	Self-identified as TG	1:77	1.300

3.2.3 FTM Transsexualism Population Frequencies

A summary of population frequency studies for FTM transsexualism is shown in Table 3.3. Studies of the population frequencies of FTM TG follow a similar pattern to those of MTF TS except that the frequencies are consistently lower and there is no research contribution from Conway and the engineers. The frequencies are at least half those of the MTF studies but over the years, the frequencies are trending upwards.

Because of the diversity of the design of these studies, it is impractical to conduct a thorough meta-analysis combining all of the results. By inspection, a conservative rule of thumb is that FTM transsexualism frequency is about half of the MTF transsexualism frequency or 0.05%.

3.2.4 FTM Transgenderism Population Frequencies

A summary of population frequency studies for FTM transgenderism is shown in Table 3.4. It is striking that the number of studies is so small. From the Zucker, Bradley, and Sanikani (1997) and Kuyper and Wijsen (2013) surveys, it appears that dissatisfaction with assigned sex and gender behavior categories is stronger among females than males. Female TGs can wear male clothing without any cultural penalties, so there is no need for formal support groups, as there seems to be with MTF transgenderism. Because of the diversity of the design of such studies, it is impractical to conduct a thorough meta-analysis, but by inspection we will set the lower bound population rule of thumb statistic as .5%, for FTM transgenderism frequency.

In conclusion, conservative population frequency estimates can be set by referencing the available data. Because of the diversity of the design of these studies, it is impractical to conduct a thorough meta-analysis combining results. Using survey and estimation approaches for the purposes of this book, we will set a best conservative estimate of MTF transsexualism as 0.1% of the male population (MTF) and for MTF transgenderism, the estimate is at least 1%. For FTM, a conservative estimate is that at least 0.05% of the female population (MTF) is transsexual, and at least 0.5% of the female population is transgender. FTM population frequencies are more difficult to estimate than MTF TS GPS. It is culturally acceptable for women to wear clothing designed for men, and their participation in support groups is lower than MTF.

3.3 SIGNIFICANCE OF POPULATION FREQUENCY ESTIMATES

The current estimated population frequencies for TSTG are several orders of magnitude higher than earlier estimates. These previous estimates were based on clinic intake and attendance criteria rather than mathematical estimates or surveys.

Table 3.3. Summary of population frequency studies for female-to-male transsexualism. *Note:* Eklund et al. reference is for reports for 1980 and 1986. FTM = female-to-male; GPS = genital plastic surgery; HT = hormone therapy; MTF = male-to-female; postop = postoperative; TS = transsexualism.

Year	Author(s)	Location	TG/TS	Type	MTF/FTM	Criterion	Odds	Percent
1968	Walinder	Sweden	TS	Clinical diagnosis	FTM		1:103000	0.0010
1968	Pauly	World	TS	Postop	FTM		1:400000	0.0003
1974	Hoenig & Kenna	England/Wales	TS	Clinical diagnosis	FTM		1:108000	0.0009
1980	Eklund et al.	Netherlands	TS	HT	FTM		1:100000	0.0010
1981	Ross, et al.	Australia	TS	Clinical	FTM	Psychiatrist survey	1:150000	0.0007
1986	Eklund et al.	Netherlands	TS	HT	FTM		1:54000	0.0019
1993	Bakker et al.	Netherlands	TS	Diagnosed TS	FTM		1:30000	0.0033
1996	Weitze & Osburg	Germany	TS	Passport change	FTM		1:104000	0.0010
1996	van Kesteren et al.	Netherlands	TS	Clinical	FTM		1:30400	0.0033
1998	Tsoi	Singapore	TS	Seeking surgery	FTM		1:8300	0.0120
1999	Wilson et al.	Scotland	TS	Hormones	FTM	TS HT	.64/100000	0.0006
1999	Wilson et al.	Scotland	TS	Postop	FTM	TS Postop	1.28/100000	0.0013

(Continued)

Table 3.3. (*Continued*)

Year	Author(s)	Location	TG/TS	Type	MTF/FTM	Criterion	Odds	Percent
2006	Gómez Gil et al.	Spain	TS	Clinical diagnosis	FTM		1:48096	0.0021
2007	DeCupere et al.	Belgium	TS	Postop	FTM		1:33800	0.0030
2008	Horton	United States	TS	Postop	FTM	U.S. GPS MD Survey	1:4200	0.0238
2008	Horton	United States	TS	Preop	FTM	U.S. GPS MD Survey	1:1400	0.0714
2008	Veale	New Zealand	TS	Passport change	FTM		1:22174	0.0045
2010	Brain	Austrailia	TS	Passport change	FTM		1:5000	0.0200

Table 3.4. Summary of population frequency studies for female-to-male transgenderism. FTM = female-to-male; GID = gender identity disorder; GLBT = gay, lesbian, bisexual, and transgender; MTF = male-to-female; TG = transgenderism.

Year	Author(s)	Location	TG/TS	Type	MTF/FTM ratio	Criterion	Odds	Percent
1997	Zucker et al.	Canada	TG	Would prefer to be opposite sex	FTM	Children	1:28	3.5000
1999	Wilson et al.	Scotland	TG	Clinical intake	FTM	No treatment	.76/100000	0.0008
1999	Wilson et al.	Scotland	TG	Counseling	FTM	GID counseling	.53/100000	0.0005
2003	Coolidge et al.	United States	TG	Twin study GID ratings	Combined	Recruited by newspaper	2.3:100	2.3000
2004	Bye et al.	US: California	TG	GLBT tobacco phone survey	Combined	Lower bound	1:50	2.0000
2005	Langstrom & Zucker	Sweden	TG	Clinical	FTM	Survey TG aroused	1:25000	0.0040
2005	van Beijsterveldt et al.	Netherlands	TG	Twins at 7 years old	FTM	Cross gender behavior by mothers	1:19	5.2000
2005	van Beijsterveldt et al.	Netherlands	TG	Twins at 10 years old	FTM	Cross gender behavior by mothers	1:30	3.3000
2008	Horton	United States	TG	Clinical GID	FTM		1:2800	0.0357
2011	Gates	United States	TG	Review of surveys	Combined		0.27291667	0.3000
2012	Clark et al.	New Zealand	TG	Youth Survey	FTM		1:83	1.2000

(Continued)

Table 3.4. (*Continued*)

Year	Author(s)	Location	TG/TS	Type	MTF/FTM ratio	Criterion	Odds	Percent
2012	Conron et al.	US: Massachusetts	TG	Health survey	Combined	Lower bound	1:250	0.4000
2012	Kuyper	Netherlands	TG	Gender identity incongruent	FTM		1:125	0.8000
2012	Kuyper	Netherlands	TG	Ambiguous about gender identity	FTM		1:31	3.2000
2013	Shields et al.	United States	TG	Middle school survey	Combined		1:77	1.3000

Population estimates have both scientific and practical significance. From a scientific point of view, the results of scientific studies can be interpreted more accurately by comparing population frequencies with those observed in such studies. From a practical point of view, it allows prediction of the capabilities and policies required to provide various services to transsexual and transgender people in the future. For example, the number of medical providers who deal with the particular problems faced by transsexual and transgender people may need to be increased. To their credit, the Great Britain and Scotland have commissioned surveys to estimate future government resources necessary to treat TSTG. As we shall see in the next chapter, professional associations for medical providers have gotten the message to their members and now encourage education in both institutions of higher learning and in continuing education. These organizations have also issued guidelines to tell doctors how to approach the doctor-patient relationship for transsexual and transgender patients.

3.4 SUMMARY

Definitions of terms for this book were developed based on biopsychological methods; these terms can serve as tools for understanding TSTG across the various scientific disciplines. Modern population frequencies for TSTG are several orders of magnitude higher than earlier estimates indicated. This is attributable to the expansion of study populations from clinical patients to large population surveys.

REFERENCES

Bakker, A., van Kestern, P. J., Gooren, L. J., & Bezemer, P. D. (1993, April). The prevalence of transsexualism in the Netherlands. *Acta Psychiatrica Scandinavica, 87*, 237–238.

Benjamin, H. (1999). *The transsexual phenomena* [online version]. Dusseldorf: Symposium Publishing (original work published 1966). Retrieved March 23, 2014, from http://www.sexarchive.info/ECE6/html/benjamin

Blanchard, R. (1989, October). The concept of autogynephilia and the typology of male gender dysphoria. *Journal of Nervous and Mental Disorders, 177*, 616–623.

Bradley, S. J., Oliver, G. D., Chernick, A. B., & Zucker, K. J. (1998). Experiment of nurture: Ablatio penis at 2 months, sex reassignment at 7 months and a psychosexual follow-up in young adulthood. *Pediatrics, 102*(1), e9.

Brain, Z. E. (2010, June 10). Prevalence of transsexuality in Australia. Retrieved July 4, 2013, from http://aebrain.blogspot.com/2010/06/prevalance-of-transsexuality-in.html.

Buhrich, N. (1978). Motivation for cross-dressing in heterosexual transvestism. *Acta Psychiatrica Scandinavica, 57,* 145–152.

Bye, L., Gruskin, E., Greenwood, G., Albright, V., & Krotki, K. (2004). *California lesbians, gays, bisexuals and transgender (LGBT) Tobacco Use Survey.* California Department of Health Services. Retrieved February 7, 2014, from http://www.cdph.ca.gov/programs/tobacco/Documents/CTCP -LGBTTobaccoStudy.pdf.

Cauldwell, D. (1949). Psychopathia transsexualis. *Sexology, 16,* 274–280.

Chivers, M., & Bailey, J. (2000). Sexual orientation of female-male transsexuals: A comparison of homosexual and nonhomosexual types. *Archives of Sexual Behavior, 29*(3), 259–278.

Clark, T., et al. (2013). *Youth'12 overview: The health and wellbeing of New Zealand secondary school students in 2012.* The University of Auckland. Retrieved April 20, 2014, from http://www.hiirc.org.nz/page/41071.

Colapinto, J. (2006). *As nature made him: The boy who was raised as a girl.* New York: Harper Perennial.

Conron, K. J., Scott, B., Stowell, G. S., & Landers, S. J. (2012). Transgender health in Massachusetts. *American Journal of Public Health, 102,* 118–122.

Conway, L. (2001–2002). *How frequently does transsexualism occur?* Retrieved July 2013 from http://www.lynnconway.com.

Coolidge, F. L., Thede, L. L., & Young, S. E. (2002). The heritability of gender identity disorder in a child and adolescent twin sample. *Behavioral Genetics, 32,* 251–257.

Costello, C. (2012, March 13). *How common is intersex status?* Accessed November 2013 from http://intersexroadshow.blogspot.com.

De Cuypere, G., Van Hemelrijck, M., Michel, A., Carael, B., Heylens, G., Rubens, R., . . . Monstrey, S. (2007, April). Prevalence and demography of transsexualism in Belgium. *European Psychiatry, 22,* 137–141.

Diamond, M., & Beh, H. (2008, January). Changes in the management of children with intersex conditions. *National Clinical Practice of Endocrinology and Metabolism, 4*(1), 4–5.

Eklund, P., Gooren, L., & Bezemer, P. (1998, May). Prevalence of transsexualism in the Netherlands. *British Journal of Psychiatry, 152,* 638–640.

Gates, G. (2011, April). *How many people are LGBT?* Williams Institute. Retrieved March 23, 2014, from http://williamsinstitute.law.ucla.edu/wp -content/uploads/Gates-How-Many-People-LGBT-Apr-2011.pdf.

Gizewski, E., Krause, E., Schlamann, M., Happich, F., Ladd, M. E., Forsting, M., & Senf, W. (2009, February). Specific cerebral activation due to visual erotic stimuli in male-to-female transsexuals compared with male and female controls: An fMRI study. *The Journal of Sexual Medicine, 6,* 440–448.

Gizewski, E. R., Krause, E., Wanke, I., Forsting, M., & Senf, W. (2006, January). Gender-specific cerebral activation during cognitive tasks using functional MRI. *Neuroradiology, 48,* 14–20.

Gómez Gil, E., Trilla García, A., Godás Sieso, T., Halperin Rabinovich, I., Puig Domingo, M., Vidal Hagemeijer, A., Peri Nogués, J. M. (2006). Estimation of prevalence, incidence and sex ratio of transsexualism in Catalonia according to health care demand [in Spanish]. *Actas Españolas de Psiquiatría, 34,* 295–302.

Hoenig, J., & Keena, C. (1974). The prevalence of transsexualism in England and Wales. *British Journal of Psychiatry, 124,* 181–190.

Horton, M. (2008). *The prevalence of SRS among US residents.* Out and Equal Workplace Summit. Retrieved February 7, 2014, from http://www.tgender.net/taw/thbcost.html.

Johannesson, L. (2014, February). *Uterine transplantation.* Presented at the 2013 WPATH Symposium, Bangkok, Thailand.

Kelly, D. (2001). *Estimation of the prevalence of transsexualism in the UK.* Retrieved February 7, 2014, from http://ai.eecs.umich.edu/people/conway/TS/UK-TSprevalence.html.

Ku, H., Lin, C. S., Chao, H. T., Tu, P. C., Li, C. T., Cheng, C. M., . . . Hsieh, J. C. (2013). Brain signature characterizing the body-brain-mind axis of transsexuals. *PLoS ONE, 8,* e70808.

Kuyper, L., & Wijsen, C. (2013). Gender identities and gender dysphoria in the Netherlands. *Archives of Sexual Behavior, 43,* 377–385.

Langstrom, N., & Zucker, K. (2005, March). Transvestic fetishism in the general population: Prevalence and correlates. *Journal of Sex and Marital Therapy, 32,* 87–95.

Morgan. (2012). Intersex in Australia. Organisation International Australia Ltd. Retrieved February 7, 2014, from http://oiiaustralia.com/author/morgan.

Oliven, J. (1965, June). Transgenderism = transsexualism. *Sexual Hygiene and Pathology,* 514.

Olyslager, F., & Conway, L. (2007, September). *On the calculation of the prevalence of transsexualism.* Presented at the 2007 WPATH Symposium, Chicago, IL.

Paoletti, J. (2012). *Pink and blue: Telling the boys from the girls in America.* Bloomington: Indiana University Press.

Pauly, I. (1968, November). The current status of the change of sex operation. *Journal of Nervous and Mental Disease, 147,* 460–471.

Pearson, G. (1996, October). Of sex and gender. *Science, 18,* 324–329.

Prince, V. (1976). Transgenderism. *Transvestia Magazine.*

Raya-Rivera, A. M., Esquiliano, D., Fierro-Pastrana, R., López-Bayghen, E., Valencia, P., Ordorica-Flores, R., . . . Atala, A. (2014, April 11). Tissue-engineered autologous vaginal organs in patients: A pilot cohort study [published online ahead of print]. *The Lancet.* doi:10.1016 /S0140-6736(14)60542-0.

Reed, B., Rhodes, S., Schofield, P., & Wylie, K. (2008, September). *Gender variance: Prevalence and trend.* Presented at the LGBTI Health Summit, London, England.

Reed, B., Rhodes, S., Schofield, P., & Wylie, K. (2009). *Gender variance in the UK: Prevalence, incidence, growth and geographic distribution.* GIRES.

Reiner, W., & Gearhart, J. (2004, January). Discordant sexual identity in some genetic males with cloacal exstrophy assigned to female sex at birth. *The New England Journal of Medicine, 350,* 333–431.

Ross, M., Walinder, J., Lundstrom, B., & Thuwe, J. (1981). Cross-cultural approaches to transsexualism. *Acta Psychiatrica Scandinavica, 63,* 75–82.

Schöning, S., Engelien, A., Bauer, C., Kugel, H., Kersting, A., Roestel, C., . . . Konrad, C. (2010, May). Neuroimaging differences in spatial cognition between men and male-to-female transsexuals before and during hormone therapy. *Journal of Sexual Medicine, 7,* 1858–1867.

Shields, J. P., Cohen, R., Glassman, J. R., Whitaker, K., Franks, H., & Bertolini, I. (2013). Estimating population size and demographic characteristics of lesbian, gay, bisexual, and transgender youth in middle school. *Journal of Adolescent Health, 53,* 248–250.

Stoller, R. (1964). A contribution to the study of gender identity. *Int. J. Psycho. 45,* 220–226.

Tsoi, W. (1988, October). The prevalence of transsexualism in Singapore. *Acta Psychiatrica Scandinavica, 78,* 502–504.

Van Beijsterveldt, C., Hudziak, J., & Boomsma, D. (2006). Genetic and environmental influences on cross-gender behavior and relation to behavior problems: A study of Dutch twins at ages 7 and 10 years. *Archives of Sexual Behavior, 35,* 647–658.

van Kesteren, P., Gooren, L., & Megens, J. (1996, December). An epidemiological and demographic study of transsexuals in the Netherlands. *Archives of Sexual Behavior, 25,* 589–600.

Veale, J. (2008). The prevalence of transsexualism among New Zealand passport holders. *Australian and New Zealand Journal of Psychiatry, 42,* 887–889.

Walinder, J. (1968). Transsexualism: Definition, prevalence and sex distribution. *Acta Psychiatrica Scandinavica Supplement, 203,* 255–258.

Waterlow, L. (2013, June 10). Too much in the pink! *Mail Online.* Retrieved February 7, 2014, from http://www.dailymail.co.uk/femail/article-2338976 /Too-pink-How-toys-alarmingly-gender-stereotyped-Seventies--cost -little-girls-self-esteem.html.

Weitze, C., & Osburg, S. (1996, August). Transsexualism in Germany: Empirical data on epidemiology and application of the German Transsexual's Act during its first ten years. *Archives of Sexual Behavior, 25,* 409–425.

Wilson, P., Sharp, C., & Carr, S. (1999, December). The prevalence of gender dysphoria in Scotland: A primary care study. *British Journal of General Practice, 49,* 991–992.

Winter, S. (2002). Counting Kathoey. *Transgender Asia Papers, 27.* Retrieved February 7, 2014, from http://web.hku.hk/~sjwinter/TransgenderASIA /paper_counting_kathoey.htm.

Zucker, K., Bradley, S., & Sanikani, M. (1997, June). Sex differences in referral rates of children with gender identity disorder. *Journal of Abnormal Child Psychology, 25,* 217–227.

4

Historical and Contemporary Cultures

4.0 INTRODUCTION

The binary gender system consists of two gender behavior categories, masculine and feminine. It is the predominant gender system among the cultures of today. However, many cultures have constructed gender systems with more than two gender behavior categories. Such gender systems have existed both historically and today. They have existed all over the world. These cultures created multiple gender behavior categories and assigned children to these categories based on criteria such as natal sex, early behavior, and expressions of gender identity. In many of these nonbinary cultures, people moved freely between gender behavior categories, depending on individual and societal needs. When they moved between gender categories, they adopted the presentation and dress rules and norms of that category.

With this backdrop of diversity in gender behavior categories, transsexualism and transgenderism (TSTG) can be seen as an attempt by people with a biological gender predisposition to find a congruent gender behavior category. Both transsexualism and transgenderism are terms that arose in the latter half of the 20th century to reflect people who violated cultural rules to follow their congruent gender behavior categories. In the contemporary binary gender system, the number of behavior categories available is limited to two and, unlike other gender systems, the current binary system is intolerant of movement from one gender behavior category to another.

It should be noted that there are reasons for cross-dressing that fall outside of the contemporary TSTG definition. Historically and even today, cross-dressing may be motivated by factors other than gender predisposition including theatrics, politics, adventure, religion, publicity, economics, and necessity. For example, males appeared in drag in plays at the time of Shakespeare because women were prohibited by culture from acting. The term **drag** seems to have been derived from theater slang for "dressed as a girl." In today's culture, cross-dressing is acceptable for drag queen and drag king performers, although most performers are not transsexual or transgender. Some are gay males and some are even natal females. Drag is often used for other purposes, such as in political protests to call attention to a cause. Historically, some females have dressed as men to go into the military in pursuit of adventure when military service was only granted for males.

4.1 ANTIQUITY

The earliest scientific evidence for movement between gender behavior categories was discovered outside of Prague in 2011 at burial sites from the Corded Ware culture of the Copper Age (2900–2500 BCE, Geen, 2011). For this culture, burial rules were strict and required a male to be buried with weapons facing to the West and a female buried with jugs facing to the East. However, archaeologists found one male buried with jugs facing to the East and one female buried with weapons facing toward the West. We know that this culture would not make such mistakes given the reverence they held for the dead, perhaps indicating that there were more than two genders in the culture or that people were allowed to move between gender behavior categories.

Another example in antiquity that is often cited in history books is that of the cross-dressing behavior of Queen Hatshepsut of Egypt (Brown, 2009) who ruled from 1479 to 1458 BCE. Although female, Hatshepsut presented in masculine clothing, including pharaoh's headdress, kilt, and the false beard associated with males. She was represented in statues and texts with a male presentation. It is not clear whether she cross-dressed because she had a gender predisposition toward a masculine gender behavior category or whether it was a political performance to maintain power.

There are numerous reports in antiquity of eunuchs who were voluntarily castrated. Becoming a eunuch frequently brought increased economic and social advantages including promotion to courtier, harem manager, and government office. Later in history, boy singers were castrated to maintain their child soprano/contralto voices. They were called *castrati*. Castrati were accepted by various cultures and religious cultures from antiquity until the mid-19th century. The tradition holds that these boys gave their informed consent for castration, although today we would not accept consent from minors as being valid. Because they had incentives to get castrated or were coerced, it is not fair to equate eunuch and *castrati* motivations with contemporary transsexual and transgender motivations.

4.2 NORTH AMERICAN NATIVE AMERICAN CULTURES

North American Native American cultures were highly diverse with respect to gender behavior categories. Anthropologists obtained detailed knowledge of these categories before the cultures were completely disrupted by the encroachment of Western culture. The names and behaviors of these gender behavior categories were captured, and there are a great many tribes that went beyond the binary system. Our current knowledge of these cultures supports the idea that the Native Americans acknowledged the need for alternatives to deal with diverse gender predispositions. Children were channeled into gender behavior categories on the basis of their early behavior as well as their natal sex.

North American Native cultures provided multiple gender behavior categories (Roscoe, 2000). In more than 100 tribes, there were three categories: there were masculine and feminine categories that were based on natal sex, and a third category that included males assuming the feminine gender role. More than 50 tribes had four categories with the addition of the category of females assuming masculine gender roles. The tribes had names for these roles. Some applied to males assuming the feminine role such as Lakota *winkte* or Ojibwa *agokwa,* and others applied to females assuming the masculine role such as Mojave *hwame* and Sauk *ickoue.* Some applied to both third and fourth gender behavior categories such as Navajo *nadleehi* and Northern Paiute *tubas.* These third and fourth gender behavior categories differed from the masculine and feminine categories in presentation and social behavior. They were believed to have special spiritual gifts and served as healers in many tribes. Some formed same-sex relations with people of masculine and feminine behavior categories. The North American tribes with alternative gender roles were geographically dispersed but primarily in what are now the Western continental United States, Canada, Alaska, and Mexico. There are some records of such alternative gender roles in South America, but the evidence is scant.

Many of the native tribes of North America followed the **two-spirit** tradition, which means that person experienced inspiration from two spirits to behave in two gender behavior categories. The story of the two-spirit tradition began in childhood. If children demonstrated gender behavior that was contrary to the usual behavior category assigned to their sex, then the tribes recognized such children as two-spirit, meaning that they possessed two transcendental, ethereal spirits (Williams, 1924/1986). For those children designated two-spirit, the tribes encouraged movement between multiple gender behavior categories. Their upbringing involved training on the skills of different gender behavior categories. For example, such children may have been taught the warrior skills consistent with one behavior category and were also taught weaving and crafts consistent with a different behavior category.

The most famous two-spirit was probably We'Wha, a Zuni who traveled to Washington in 1886 to meet President Grover Cleveland and to show her handicraft arts and culture to him. She was celebrated as an artisan in weaving, pottery, and blanket making (Roscoe, 2000). She took pride in her child rearing and domestic skills. She stood six feet tall and wore feminine clothing. It was only after she left Washington that it was revealed that she was an *lhamana*, a male assuming the feminine gender role. But We'Wha also sometimes assumed the role of male warrior as needed and was credited with many kills in battle.

According to the two-spirit tradition when these children became adults, they would assume important positions in the tribe because of their varied insight, spirituality, and experience. Such two-spirit adults presented themselves in whatever gender behavior category was appropriate without regard to their natal sex. Some became mediators, artisans, medicine men, or shamans; others became chiefs. It is believed that some famous Native American tribal chiefs had nicknames indicating their two-spirit status.

Sexual orientation of two-spirit individuals varied, and they were allowed to form permanent same-sex associations. Because two-spirits had such valuable skills, the partner or "spouse" of a two-spirit would achieve greater status within the tribe and achieve greater prosperity. Some two-spirits even simulated menstrual cycles by cutting themselves in the groin to bleed to validate their claim to a feminine gender behavior category.

Two-spirits have been termed *berdache* according to the term used by the Spanish invaders for young male homosexual prostitutes. The term was borrowed from the Persian through Muslim Spain. This pejorative name betrayed the Spanish lack of understanding of the Native American culture and assumed that those with alternative gender roles were homosexual prostitutes. It is believed that neither the Native Americans themselves nor the anthropologists, who initially popularized it, actually knew the origin of the name berdache. In the early 1990s, a group of Native American anthropologists and leaders adopted the term *two-spirit* and urged that other scientists do the same.

The term two-spirit recently underwent yet another evolution in meaning due to Native Americans reclaiming their heritage. It now is sometimes used to refer to all Native American gay, lesbian, bisexual, transgender, and queer people. One has to determine if the term is used in this way by context or by inquiry because it is different from traditional scientific usage.

Surprisingly, one Native American culture still exists that has a third gender behavior category in its essential form, as far as can be determined. This is the male-to-female (MTF) *muxe* of southern Mexico who claim heritage to the Zapotec tribe. Remnants of the Native American Zapotec tribe still exist although the tribe was nearly obliterated by Spanish invasions in the 15th to

17th centuries (Lacey, 2008). *Muxe* are publicly accepted by the communities in the remote towns of Oaxaca and Juchitán near the border between Mexico and Guatemala. They cross-dress, and some take hormones. Annual festivals in these towns celebrate the *muxe*. The *muxe* fit within the contemporary MTF TSTG concepts, even though their culture is centuries old. The survival of the *muxe* tradition was probably due to the relative isolation of this area of Mexico.

4.3 CONTEMPORARY WESTERN TSTG

The contemporary Western model of TSTG began in the mid-20th century with the concepts of transexualism and transgenderism. As we saw in Chapter 3, transsexuals and transgender people are not rare. Based mainly on Western sources, the population frequency of transgender male to female is at least 1%, and for transsexual males, it is at least .1% (see Section 3.2 and 3.3). Female-to-male (FTM) frequencies are about one half of those for MTF, although obtaining accurate estimates is difficult for FTM because culture allows them to dress in a wide range of fashion.

Although castration had been practiced back into antiquity, transsexualism began with the modern plastic surgical capability to change male genitalia to look more like female genitalia. The procedures were pioneered and perfected in Germany, the United Kingdom, Sweden, and Denmark and later in the United States. The first practical operating techniques were developed in the United Kingdom during the 1940s. Christine Jorgenson became the first widely known transsexual through surgeries in Denmark and the United States. In 1972, Sweden became the first country to pass laws regarding the surgeries and granted transsexuals the rights and obligations of their new legal sex assignment. Transition procedures became standardized for transsexuals by the Harry Benjamin International Gender Dysphoria Association, later renamed the World Professional Association for Transgender Health.

Starting in the 1960s, the term *transgender* became popular in the United States and has now spread throughout the world. It originally referred to those who cross-dressed full time without body changes, although some transgender people in that era did take hormones. The word *transgender* was used in place of transvestite to deemphasize the role that sexual arousal played in cross-dressing. Transgender has now become an umbrella term for all who do not conform to the gender behavior category that they were assigned at birth and conform to a different gender behavior category, either part or full time. Although many perform their TSTG behavior in private, many eventually come out of the closet at least as far as attending support groups or visiting TSTG-friendly public establishments.

As long ago as the mid-20th century, connecting to other transsexual or transgender people was difficult. Informal cross-dressing groups did meet in secret in the United States and elsewhere, but locating one was difficult and risky. We do know that such groups existed from photographs and histories. Typically, a group of cross-dressers would rent a secluded house for weekends or found locations in large cities.

It was difficult to find out about TSTG or reach out to others until transsexual and transgender people built up a network of support groups during the 1960s modeled after other support groups. The 1970s were the heyday of support group formation for such issues as civil rights, self-help, and human rights as well as TSTG. The model for these support groups was Alcoholics Anonymous, started in 1935, but unlike the Alcoholics Anonymous model the purpose of these transgender support groups was to encourage rather than discourage behavior. Cross-dressing support groups were featured in national magazines. These groups allowed transsexuals and transgender people to obtain peer-group counseling and information and make social contacts. The format of the transgender support groups usually encourages participants to go out after meetings with support group participants to known safe bars and restaurants. Most transgender people do not stay in the support group permanently but find that they can rely on their new social contacts for support. Some stay on to help other transgender people.

TSTG support groups exist all over the United States and the world. Some are independent; others are affiliated with networks of support groups such as the Society for the Second Self (known as Tri-Ess), which was started by activist Virginia Prince, who also published the magazine *Transvestia* from 1960 to 1980. Some support groups still require interviews before a TSTG can be admitted for the sake of privacy, and some groups are transgender or heterosexual only or require attendance of a significant other. Tri-Ess is strictly a heterosexual group that seeks to involve significant others and their families. Other support groups are open to anyone who thinks that they are transsexual or transgender or genderqueer. Some pansexual TSTG groups are also open to gay and bisexual people who may be TSTG as well and are trying to figure out both their sexual orientation and their gender behavior category.

Computer "bulletin boards" provided connectivity for transsexual and transgender people in the 1970s and 1980s until the Internet became available. Closed computer network social connections had a side benefit because TSTG had some hope of maintaining their privacy, unlike the Internet.

In the late 1980s, the International Foundation for Gender Education provided educational information and listings of support groups and conferences in their magazine *Tapestry*. This provided a guide for transsexual and transgender people to seek support, help, mental health counseling, and companionship. In particular, it advertised TSTG conferences where TSTG could cross-dress in safety for longer periods of time. These conferences continue today all across the United States and the United Kingdom. The largest of which is Southern Comfort in Atlanta, which draws 1,000 to 1,200 transsexuals and transgender people, both MTF and FTM, annually with educational seminars and social events. Significant others also attend and Southern Comfort also typically includes a track of presentations and workshops for them.

The Western contemporary model for TSTG practices was not derived directly from historical cultures. However, it is known that cross-dressers did exist in the West in earlier times, predating the modern TSTG models. There are numerous stories about transgender people in Europe and the United States, many of whom were engaged in high visibility, sometimes flamboyant activities including politics, the military (Terris, 2013), settling the United States Western frontier, and espionage. The names of these people include the Chevalier d'Eon, a French diplomat and spy; Henry Hyde, Viscount Cornbury, British governor of New York and New Jersey (Devor, 1996); Mary/Mark Red, a Caribbean pirate; and Albert Cashier, Union solder in the U.S. Civil War (Terris, 2013). More recently they include Billie Tipton, an American musician; Charley Parkhurst, stagecoach driver and early California settler; Ed Wood, movie director; and Jan Morris, author. It is not clear that the motivation of these people was to find a congruent gender behavior category, except for Jan Morris who wrote about it extensively in her autobiography (1974).

Transsexuals and transgender people are legally protected from workplace and public accommodation discrimination in many European countries and in a handful of states in the United States. Discrimination is still de facto practiced in some European countries, especially in Eastern Europe and United States localities with strong fundamentalist feelings. Sterilization is required as well as TS genital plastic surgery (GPS) in 8 of 15 Eastern European countries.

Most of the scientific research on TSTG is conducted in European countries such as the Netherlands and the United Kingdom as a sidelight of clinical practice. Some research is carried out in Australia, New Zealand, and Canada. Research in the United States has been confined mainly to applied research aimed at improving TSTG public health, especially involving eradication of HIV/AIDS and other diseases.

4.4 ASIAN CULTURES AND PACIFIC OCEAN

There are many historical peoples in Pacific Ocean and Asian cultures who had alternate gender categories. Few of these survive today. Most of their cultures were disrupted by colonization (Jaffrey, 1996), religious missionaries, and infiltration by modern Western culture. The largest group that survives is the *hijra* of South Asia, who maintain they are a "third sex." The most visible contemporary group in this area of the world is the *kathoey* of Thailand. The transgender *waria* of Indonesia recently achieved visibility when it was reported that Barak Obama had had a waria nanny as a child. There are contemporary transsexual and transgender people reported in most countries, but acceptance varies widely.

The *hijra* are a third-sex subculture based mainly in India and neighboring countries. Estimates of the *hijra* population vary widely between 130,000 to several million. The problem with getting accurate estimates is that many are counted in censuses and surveys as either male or female. This situation will change soon in that India and other countries that are making more precise surveys and providing a third gender category marker for identification cards (Haider, 2009). *Hijra* include MTF transgender, MTF transsexual, intersex, and some natal females. They are rejected by the larger societies and are regarded as being in the lowest socioeconomic class. *Hijra* see themselves as a third sex and practice a third gender category (Nanda, 1999). They are discriminated against with regard to employment, which traditionally limited them to begging, performing at birth celebrations, performing at weddings, and prostitution. Some have now managed to find more respectable careers. *Hijra* trace their heritage back at least 500 years in relation to worship of the Hindu god Vishnu, although they now practice many religions. They are organized into communal families with a guru leader who collects intelligence on local fund-raising opportunities, regulates member dress and behavior, and coordinates family activities. Indian gurus report to one of seven *najak* leaders who run the seven *hijra* "houses." *Hijra* perform *nirvan* castrations on their members, but most members are nontranssexual transgender people. *Hijra* have become politically active, and several hold elective office.

Unlike the *hijra*, the *kathoey* of Thailand are for the most part accepted in their country and culture. A behavioral observation survey indicated that there were more than 17,000 *kathoey* in Bangkok alone (Winter & Udomsak, 2002) and upward of 180,000 in the whole country. *Kathoey* are MTF transsexuals and transgender people who regard themselves as a "second category of females" and believe that their TSTG is biological. They present in feminine clothing, makeup, vocabulary, and voice (Winter & Udomsak, 2002). Many of them take hormones, and some get TS GPS and breast enhancement surgery. They also participate in beauty contests for *kathoey* in Thailand. The *kathoey* mainly participate in the sex trade although they are gradually assuming other occupations including teaching, retail sales, and entertainment. Some hide their transsexualism or transgenderism while on the job during working hours. Religions in Thailand bless marriages between males and *kathoey*, although the marriages do not have legal status.

The *waria* of Indonesia gathered worldwide attention in 2012 after a story was published about the plight of Barack Obama's nanny (Associated Press, 2012). Obama's mother, Ann Dunham, did sociological research in Indonesia, and while she was there, she hired a nanny, Evie, who was a *waria*, for Barack. After Obama's family left, Evie fell on hard times. She subsequently became unemployed and became a sex worker and a victim of violence.

Waria are MTF transgender people who refuse to feminize their bodies because of religious belief but present in the feminine gender behavior category (Huffington Post, 2012). There are an estimated 7 million *waria* in Indonesia out of a population of 240 million. They are highly visible in Indonesian society and participate openly in the beauty and entertainment industries. However, there is still lingering cultural rejection of *waria* by Indonesia culture. Many have positions in respected businesses but hide the fact that they are *waria*. There are organized *waria* beauty pageants at the district and national level that have achieved international recognition.

Although TSTG have largely become Westernized in most Pacific Rim countries, some native subcultures that have multiple gender categories still exist, although they are increasingly under stress. An example of a historical gender category that did not survive is the *mahu* of Hawaii, which was indigenous to the Kanak Maoli culture. The *mahu* could be either males or females and practiced a gender behavior category between masculine and feminine. They engaged in teaching and were keepers of cultural oral tradition.

The Siberian *Chuckchi* are a nomadic people who rely on reindeer for food and clothing. They have a third gender behavior category, the members of which are males who adopt feminine roles but go with males on the hunt. Although the *Chuckchi* still exist today, little is known about their third gender because of isolation. The *Chuckchi* avoid contact with contemporary culture. There was a series of unsuccessful genocidal wars by the Russians aimed at eliminating the *Chuckchi* and their culture; the last one ended with the Russian commander's head displayed on a pike.

The traditional *fa'afafine* of Samoa (Bartlett & Vasey, 2006), the *fakaleiti* of Tonga, and the *whakawahine* of New Zealand are considered third genders of males who practice feminine gender roles, including family care. They also engage in the arts, fashion, and other occupations. They are not considered homosexual by their culture, although they may engage in sexual relations with males, females, and other third-gender-category people. The *fa'afafine* have formed political organizations to try to preserve their rights and culture.

The *bakla* of the Philippines are a minority of gender-diverse people who are males who adopt feminine behavior roles and are mainly attracted to males. The *bakla* have developed their own language, which is a mixture of English, Spanish, and local dialects, and have their own stores and beauty pageants. They make voluntary body changes including taking hormones and getting breast implants, but TS GPS is rare. Although they have been embedded in the culture of the Philippines for at least several centuries, they are now under extreme cultural stress.

The Bugis people in Indonesia recognize five gender behavior categories (Graham, 2001). In addition to males and females, they have *calabai, calalai,* and *bissu*. The *calabai* are males who assume many feminine behaviors, and the *calalai* are females who assume masculine occupations and behaviors.

Bissu are "gender-transcendent" individuals who combine behaviors from masculine and feminine behavior categories; their function is to provide advice and inspiration to the culture. Traditional Islam usually does not permit nonreligious clergy such as the *bissu* to engage in activities that may compete with recognized religious leaders, but accommodations have been made through theological arguments and fatwas to tolerate *bissu* activities.

Other contemporary transsexuals and transgender people can be found in most countries in the Pacific and on the Pacific Rim. Most are according to the contemporary Western model.

4.5 MIDDLE EAST AND AFRICAN CULTURES

Most of the historical cultures in the Middle East and Africa were disrupted by colonization, war, and religious missionaries, so native culture was almost obliterated. We will never know what gender behavior categories might have been developed. In many Middle East and African countries, TSTG behavior is illegal and punishable by imprisonment or death. Reports of raids on cross-dressing groups by religious police periodically emerge from these countries (Morgan, 2014). There are two notable exceptions: the *xanith* of Oman and the transsexual policies of Iran.

The *xanith* of Oman are males who adopt feminine behavior category roles and, under local Islamic law, have the same rights as men. They do not wear the mask and veil of women, but present in a composite of masculine and feminine styles. They have sexual relations with both males and females, taking the submissive sexual role with males. They are able to marry females. Many serve as male prostitutes, but others have substantial careers.

Transgender people in Iran are subject to death or imprisonment if discovered but can avoid these penalties if they undergo transsexual transition and TS GPS. Because the Ayatollah Khomeini published a fatwa sanctioning TS GPS for transsexuals, such surgery is encouraged and is state subsidized. There is some belief that homosexuals are being coerced into transsexual transition, because they too face imprisonment and death sentences if discovered. After Thailand, the second leading country for TS GPS is Iran.

4.6 SOUTH AMERICAN CULTURES

TSTG in South America generally follows the Western contemporary model, and Argentina, Brazil, and Chile have passed laws protecting their civil rights (Garcia, 2012). All three countries support transsexual transition and TS GPS in their national health systems. However, TSTG still suffer de facto exclusion from many occupations based on cultural intolerance. Many are forced into prostitution. The rate of violence against transsexual and transgender people is highest in Brazil and continues to increase. In 2013, Brazil had the highest number of transgender murders in the world, with 95. By comparison, Brazil was followed by Mexico with 40 and the United States with 16 (Transgender Europe, 2014).

4.7 SUMMARY

Not all cultures have adopted the prevailing Western gender binary system of masculine/feminine. This chapter provides examples of cultures that have adopted multiple gender categories. Some cultures have allowed movement between gender behavior categories depending on the needs of the individual and the culture. It is likely that these cultures were responding to biological gender predispositions of their children.

The gender categories of these cultures cannot easily be equated with the concept of TSTG that came out of Western culture in the middle of the 20th century. However, the concept of biological gender predisposition does pertain to TSTG. As was noted earlier in this text, TSTG occurs when biological gender predisposition is incongruent with culturally assigned gender behavior category. In the current binary system, TSTG can choose from only two categories, masculine and feminine. In the prevailing Western culture, all people are required to follow their culturally assigned gender behavior categories, which makes transsexual and transgender people cultural outlaws.

The current Western culture views it as a cultural violation for people to move to a more congruent gender behavior category, but some cultures such as the Native American two-spirits could easily exist within such a category without violating their culture.

REFERENCES

Associated Press. (2012, March 6). Obama's transgender former nanny living in fear in Indonesia. *The Guardian*. Retrieved February 7, 2014, from http://www.theguardian.com/world/2012/mar/06/obama-former-nanny-transgender-trial-indonesia.

Bartlett, N., & Vasey, P. (2006). A retrospective study of childhood gender-atypical behavior in Samoan *fa'afafine*. *Archives of Sexual Behavior*, 35, 559–566.

Brown, C. (2009, April). The king herself. *National Geographic*. Retrieved July 4, 2013, from http://ngm.nationalgeographic.com/2009/04/hatshepsut/brown-text.

Devor, H. (1996, April). The tradition of female transvestism in early modern Europe. *Archives of Sexual Behavior*, 25, 1-144.

Garcia, P. (2012). Chilean paradoxes: LGBT rights in Latin America. *The Huffington Post*. Retrieved July 4, 2013, from http://www.huffingtonpost.

com/pedro-garcia/chilean-paradoxes-lgbt-rights-in-latin-america_b_
1819455.html.

Geen, J. (2011, April). 5,000-year-old "transgender" skeleton. *Pink News.*
Retrieved July 4, 2013, from http://www.pinknews.co.uk/2011/04/06/5000
-year-old-transgender-skeleton-discovered.

Graham, S. (2001, April). Sulawesi's fifth gender. *Inside Indonesia.*
Retrieved July 4, 2013, from http://www.insideindonesia.org/edition-66
/sulawesi-s-fifth-gender-3007484.

Haider, Z. (2009, December 23). Pakistan's supreme court ordered authorities on Wednesday to allow transvestites and eunuchs to identify themselves as a distinct gender as part of a move to ensure their rights. Reuters.
Retrieved February 7, 2014, from http://uk.reuters.com/article/2009/12/23
/us-pakistan-transvestites-idINTRE5BM2BX20091223.

Huffington Post. (2012, May 26). Tales of the *waria*: Inside Indonesia's
third-gender community. Retrieved February 7, 2014, from http://www
.huffingtonpost.com/kathy-huang/tales-of-the-waria-indonesia_b
_1546629.html.

Jaffrey, Z. (1996). *The invisibles: A tale of the eunuchs of India.* New York:
Pantheon.

Lacey, M. (2008, December 6). The *muxe* of Mexico. *New York Times.*
Retrieved February 7, 2014, from http://www.nytimes.com/2008/12/07
/weekinreview/07lacey.html?_r=0.

Morgan, J. (2014, April 9). Saudi Arabia police arrest 35 for having a "gay party."
Gay Star News. Retrieved April 12, 2014, from http://www.gaystarnews
.com/article/saudi-arabia-police-arrest-35-having-gay-party090414.

Morris, J. (1974). *Conundrum.* New York: Signet.

Nanda, S. (1999). *Neither man nor woman: The* hijras *of India.* New York:
Wadsworth. Retrieved July 4, 2013, from http://petervas.files.wordpress
.com/2013/03/serena_nanda.pdf.

Roscoe, W. (2000). *Changing ones: Third and fourth genders in native North
America.* New York: Palgrave Macmillan.

Terris, B. (2013, January 24). A history of crossdressing soldiers. *The Atlan-
tic.* Retrieved from http://www.theatlantic.com/sexes/archive/2013/01
/a-history-of-crossdressing-soldiers/272500.

Transgender Europe. (2014). *Transgender Europe's Trans Murder Monitoring
Project.* Retrieved January 31, 2014, from http://www.tgeu.org/node/435.

Williams, W. (1986). *The spirit and the flesh, sexual diversity in the American
Indian Culture.* Boston: Beacon. (Original work published 1924.)

Winter, S., & Udomsak, N. (2002). Male, female and transgender: Stereotypes and self in Thailand. *International Journal of Transgenderism,* 6(1).
Retrieved February 6, 2014, from http://www.transgenderasia.org/paper
_male_female.htm.

Genetic Causal Factor in Transsexualism and Transgenderism

5.0 INTRODUCTION

This chapter presents additional evidence to show that transsexualism and transgenderism (TSTG) is a biological phenomenon by presenting scientific results on TSTG genetics. This evidence begins to reveal the causal factors involved in TSTG. Evidence was presented in the preceding three chapters that TSTG is a biological phenomenon. In Chapter 2, the tragic case of David Reimers and other evidence indicate that there are biological gender behavior predispositions that cannot be changed by child rearing. In Chapter 3, it was demonstrated that the strength of the gender behavior predisposition is so strong that TSTG behavior persists despite rejection by parents, friends, family, community, church, and other cultural institutions. TSTG behavior persists in the face of deleterious consequences for the individual including the effects of secrecy, depression, and potential suicide. In Chapter 4, evidence demonstrated numerous gender systems with more than two gender behavior categories, indicating that some cultures adapt their gender behavior categories to the gender predispositions of its offspring. It also demonstrated the wide extent of TSTG and related phenomena that are indicative of a biological phenomenon.

Because TSTG realization emerges about age 4 years, there are three primary causal factors that could be involved in TSTG. The three candidate causal factors are genetics, epigenetics, and early child rearing. Studies of early child rearing presented in Chapter 8 indicate that this candidate causal factor can temporarily be ruled out, given current developmental psychology science results. Only two candidate causal factors remain—genetics and epigenetics. DNA genetics is a potential causal factor in biological behavioral predisposition resulting from its expression to form and regulate the brain and body. Epigenetics involves the study of mechanisms that modify DNA or change its expression, which changes the body (phenotype) of individuals or their behavior. The interactions of genetics and epigenetics as causal factors lead to the two-factor theory of TSTG causation, discussed in Chapter 7. The present chapter summarizes the evidence for DNA genetic causal factors in TSTG beginning with a brief review of relevant genetics and genetic mechanisms.

There are four lines of evidence that indicate that DNA genetics is a causal factor in TSTG. The first comes from heritability studies of twins and families. Such studies are a staple of biological and psychological inquires into the heritability of various traits. *Twin studies* measure the probability that if one identical twin has a given trait, the other twin will share that trait. "Family" heritability studies measure the correlation between various kinship states (e.g., nonidentical twins, siblings) and the family environment for a trait. From these studies, the evidence indicates that there is moderate to strong heritability for TSTG, but there is still "room" for involvement by an epigenetic factor.

The second line of evidence in the comparison of TSTG and non-TSTG DNA is to look for chromosome anomalies and marker genes that correlate with TSTG. Markers (alleles or genes) have been discovered on the DNA molecule for both male-to-female (MTF) and female-to-male (FTM) TSTG at the androgen receptor (AR) gene and a hormone metabolism gene, respectively. These markers seem to indicate some of the genes required for formation of masculine or feminine gender predispositions. However, there are probably other markers of TSTG that have yet to be found because a full scan of DNA has not yet been done for TSTG. In the past, a full DNA or genome scan was time consuming and was costly, but that has changed with the rapid advances in genetics technology. The importance of a full scan is that multiple genes working together govern many traits; for example, eye color has at least five genes that contribute to the outcome in humans (Liu et al., 2009).

The third line of evidence is that the marker for MTF transsexualism involves the **androgen receptor** (AR) gene, which is also associated with allele variations or mutations in **androgen insensitivity syndrome** (AIS). AIS is a difference in sexual development that results in female sex characteristics even though the person may have 46,XY chromosomes, which normally results in male sex characteristics. Allele variations of the AR gene are associated with cases of AIS. It is interesting that 46,XY AIS do not exhibit increases in masculine behavior that one would expect if gender predisposition were determined by genetics alone. One would expect that males with AIS would find the masculine gender behavior category to be more congruent. As was described earlier, an allele or variant of the AR gene is a marker for formation of a feminine gender predisposition. In the case of AIS, it appears that AR mutations create a feminine gender predisposition as well as preventing the effects of androgens on development. Feminine gender predisposition would be congruent with a feminine gender behavior category to which most 46,XY are assigned and thus TSTG behavior would not occur.

The fourth line of evidence is that FTM TSTG has particular characteristics that differ from non-FTM. These include teeth, pelvic shape, and other biometrics that are assumed to be due to genetic mechanisms. This provides further support for the genetic basis for FTM TSTG.

There are at least three feasible genetic mechanisms for TSTG. These include germ-line inheritance, de novo mutations, and multiple DNA in a single body. The classification of mechanisms between genetic and epigenetic is fuzzy. As used in this book, *genetics* refers to DNA expression, whereas *epigenetic mechanisms* refers to modification of DNA or modification of DNA expression.

5.1 GENETICS RELEVANT TO TSTG

Most cells in the human body feature a nucleus that contains DNA molecules organized into chromosomes. A person gets one version of each of the chromosomes from each of the two biological parents. DNA molecules are composed of relatively long helical double-stranded ladders that contain the DNA genetic code, or the genome. The backbones of the helices consist of sugar and phosphates with relatively strong bonds. Each rung of the ladder consists of a weak bond of two of four particular amino acids in four combinations. The rungs of the helical ladder encode the genetic information. This allows the DNA molecule to be easily "zipped" open for copying to new cells.

Patterns of these DNA ladder rungs that influence traits such as body formation and function are called **genes**. Different forms of the same gene are called alleles if they are frequent enough to be considered an important variation. Each allele typically appears in both of the two pairs of chromosomes but only one is normally expressed. Multiple genes are involved in most traits. There are approximately 20,000 to 25,000 genes in the human genome.

Most people have 23 pairs or 46 chromosomes that organize the DNA. Two of the 46 chromosomes contain the information necessary to start forming sex organs as well as other information. The other chromosomes are known as somatic chromosomes from the Greek word *soma*, which means "body." Males usually have one X chromosome and one Y chromosome, and females usually have two X chromosomes. However, there are many variations of chromosomes and genes that can result in male or female organs, so categorization of sex by the XX/XY test is not perfect. For example, the Olympics have long since abandoned categorization of sex by any XX/XY chromosome test. The information necessary to trigger the development of male sex organs is found on the Y chromosome, although somatic genes are also involved in the development process (Vilain & McCabe, 1998).

The address of DNA molecules within the chromosome follows a locating convention, which is like naming the location of a house by its city, street, and house number. For example, Xq11-12 is on the X-chromosome, on the longer part of the chromosome (termed q), at positions 11 and 12. An example for somatic gene location is 14q21-22, which means the gene is located on chromosome 14 on the longer part of the chromosome at positions 21 and 22. If the gene location were on the shorter end of the chromosome, it would be designated with the letter "p" instead of "q."

In addition to the nucleus, most human cells contain structures known as mitochondria. The genetics of mitochondria are passed on to offspring strictly through maternal familial lines. Mitochondria are the powerhouses of the cell because they manufacture chemicals that are used for energy in the entire cell. Mitochondria have their own DNA, so in addition to the genome of the cell nucleus, there is the mitochondrial genome.

Ribonucleic acid (RNA) molecules are also present in the cell. RNA is created from DNA and is similar in structure but has structural and functional differences. The "central dogma" of molecular genetics from the 1950s onward is that the role of RNA is to mediate the expression of DNA information by creating proteins that influence cell mechanisms. In contradiction to this dogma, it has been found that RNA performs many other functions.

We are just beginning to understand all of the functions that RNA mediates (Clancy, 2008), so there are types of the approximately 1,000 RNA chemical species that are not understood completely. However, we do know some of the important RNA functions:

- Gene expression or transmission of information to the cell
- Gene copying and proofreading
- Regulating other RNA
- "Gene switching," or modifying the likelihood that a particular gene will or will not be expressed

RNA is involved in several types of gene switching, including **repression bonding**, **gene promotion**, and **methylation**. In repression bonding, a repression chemical species binds to the DNA to inactivate its expression of a gene. Another type of off-switching involves binding to the DNA by methyl groups. In gene promotion, a promoter chemical binds to the DNA. Because DNA molecules spend most of their time curled up in a ball, those that are more accessible to binding will be expressed. To the extent that this gene switching occurs after conception, these mechanisms are forms of epigenetics.

DNA genes can change or mutate. Mutations can vary in size from a single allele or gene to a large part of a chromosome. Mutations that occur before conception (joining of egg and sperm) are called *germ-line* or *hereditary mutations*. Such mutations influence traits and are usually found in every cell of the body of the offspring. Such mutations can occur during conception, in which case they are called de novo mutations. Other mutations may occur after conception and are classed as epigenetic mutations. They are described Chapter 6.

There are two types of twins, identical or **monozygotic** and fraternal or **dizygotic**. Monozygotic twins start out at conception with identical DNA, whereas dizygotic twins do not, although they share the same mother and father. Although monozygotic twins start at conception with identical DNA, by the time they are born, their DNA and the expression of their DNA differs considerably (Bruder et al., 2008; Gordon et al., 2012).

5.2 HERITABILITY OF TSTG

The message in the DNA is expressed through RNA to produce body traits. The passing on of traits to offspring is termed heritability. Heritability of traits is typically studied using **twin studies** in which a given trait is correlated over many **twin pairs**. Even identical twins who share the same DNA at conception have somewhat different traits from each other because of subsequent genetic mutations and epigenetic mechanisms. There are also **family studies** that may include twins and siblings to explore heritability.

TSTG heritability is moderate to strong in twin and family studies. Studies of transsexualism and transgenderism are presented separately below. Most of these studies are derived from clinical data that may understate inheritance. Transsexuals and transgender people who never seek out help are generally not counted in clinical studies because of the reluctance of patients to report TSTG information about themselves and their families. There may also be reluctance on the part of investigators to share patient data due to HIPPA or ethical restrictions.

Table 5.1 summarizes the studies for TS heritability chronologically. It should be pointed out that the probability of identical monozygotic twins is relatively small (.04%), as is the probability of transsexualism (.01%), so transsexuals with identical twin siblings are scarce.

Studies from 1974 to the Veale study in 2010 were generally isolated reports of twins or triplets both having TS in very small numbers. The Green (2000) study with 20 subjects and 9 twin pairs was not definitive, but at the time, estimates of transsexual frequency were so low that it was assumed that

Table 5.1. Studies of transsexual heritability. FTM = female to male; MTF = male to female; TS = transsexual.

Year	Author	Type	Age	MZ/DZ	TS/TG	MTF/FTM	Number Twin Pairs	Percent
1974	Saballis et al.	Clinical encounter	Adult	MZ	TS	MTF	0	N/A
1977	Hyde & Kenna	Clinical encounter	Adult	MZ	TS	MTF	1	N/A
1985	Joyce & Ding	Clinical encounter	Adult	MZ	TS	FTM	0	N/A
2000	Green	Clinical encounter	Adult	MZ	TS	MTF/FTM	1	N/A
2000	Sadeghi	Clinical encounter	Adult	MZ	TS	FTM	1	N/A
2003	Hepp	Clinical encounter	Adult	MZ	TS	MTF	1	N/A
2006	Segal	Clinical encounter	Adult	MZ	TS	FTM	2	N/A
2007	Knobloch et al.	Clinical encounter	Adult	MZ	TS	FTM	1	N/A
2010	Gómez-Gil et al.	Clinical encounter	Adult	DZ	TS	MTF	677	1.30
2010	Gómez-Gil et al.	Clinical encounter	Adult	DZ	TS	FTM	318	0.31
2010	Gómez-Gil et al.	Clinical encounter	Adult	DZ	TS	MTF/FTM	677	0.63
2010	Veale et al.	Review clinical	Adult	MZ	TS	MTF	31	52.00
2010	Veale et al.	Review clinical	Adult	MZ	TS	FTM	27	40.00
2013	Diamond	Review clinical	Adult	MZ	TS	MTF	39	33.00
2013	Diamond	Review clinical	Adult	MZ	TS	FTM	35	23.00

transsexual twins were rare. Green therefore concluded that transsexualism could be inheritable.

The Gómez-Gil et al. (2010) study was unique in the transsexual heritability studies in that it did not concern monozygotic siblings at all. It concerned only non-twin dizygotic siblings. Of 677 MTF transsexuals, 9 were found to have a dizygotic MTF twin or 1.3%. Of 318 FTM transsexuals, 1 was found to also be FTM or .31%. Of the MTF transsexuals, two were found to have an opposite sex dizygotic sibling or .6%.

The last two studies on the list attempted to obtain larger samples by mining research reports and developing clinical data sources. The Veale, Clarke, & Lomax (2010) study managed to pull together data from 31 MTF and 27 FTM twin pairs with one or more TS twins from the literature. This resulted in a 50% rate for MTF and 40% rate for FTM that would indicate a high degree of heritability. However, some of the papers that Veale, Clarke, & Lomax used would have likely only been published if both twins were transsexuals.

The Diamond (2013) study attempted to find new data sources by reviewing old clinical data and contacting clinicians who have treated transsexuals for their statistics on transsexual twins. This increased the sample size somewhat but considered older cases in which transsexual twins may have been less forthcoming. The clinicians were asked if any of the transsexuals they were treating or had treated were part of a twin pair and, if so, how many twin pairs were both transsexuals. The results showed 33% for MTF and 23% for FTM, which indicates a moderate degree of DNA heritability when compared with our population rules of thumb of .1% for MTF and .05% for FTM.

Given the difficulties in finding transsexual twin pairs and possible reticence of one twin to reveal transsexualism of themselves or their sibling, a medium strength correlation is apparent for transsexual heritability. For example, the correlation is not as high as the heritability of body height, which is in the 60% to 80% range (Chao-Qiang, 2006), leaving room for other causal factors to influence transsexualism. (When parametric data are available, as in height correlations, a coefficient of concordance is calculated, but all we have for transsexualism is a percentage.) The other problem with these studies is that we do not know whether one identical twin was transsexual and the other transgender. We do not always know whether doctors asked if siblings of identical twins were transgender or not, and we do not know whether there were transgender twins still in the closet. Because commitment to transsexual transition is severely life changing, transgender twins may not have been willing or in a position to make this commitment. We also do not know whether nontranssexual identical twins subsequently became transsexual.

Heritability studies results for transgenderism are shown in Table 5.2. The heritability of transgenderism shown in these studies is moderate to high. These studies were conducted with data from large twin population registries in Australia, the Netherlands, and the United Kingdom. One study (Coolidge, Thede, & Young, 2002) used large-scale advertising for twins in the U.S. Midwest. Most of these studies included transgender children as subjects.

Three of these studies use a mathematical technique called structural equation modeling (SEM), which can partial out and quantify the variance due to genetic factors versus other factors from samples of both identical and fraternal twins. In this case, the more variance accounted for, the stronger the genetic heritability. SEM heritability models typically include genetic factors (A), common or shared environmental effects (C), and unique or non-shared environmental effects (E). They are thus referred to as ACE models. The results of applying SEM models are loadings ranging from −1 to +1 that reflect the variance accounted for by the particular ACE factor. In addition to the SEM model, some studies used polychoric correlations that were calculated for childhood "gender nonconformity" for each twin category. Polychoric correlations are used when the underlying data is interval data rather than ratio-scale data.

The first study on the list in Table 5.2 (Bailey, Dunne, & Martin, 2000) used twins drawn from the Australian National Health and Medical Research Twin Registry. It was a retrospective study for adults aged 17 to 50 using a behavioral checklist rating scale to rate their childhood transgender behavior. There were 312 male identical twins, 182 male fraternal twins, 376 female identical twins, and 353 opposite-sex twins. Each twin filled out a rating scale that was composed of cross-behavior and gender identity items. The intent of the authors was to establish the heritability of homosexuality but the data on homosexuality did not support this conclusion. The results of this study indicated moderate heritability for both MTF and FTM.

Results of the Bailey study for gender nonconformity for various twin categories are shown in Table 5.2. The SEM model included MTF and FTM and included all three ACE components. The genetic components of the ACE model were .5 for MTF and .64 for FTM. The polychoric correlations for MTF monozygotic twins was .45 to .65. For FTM, the correlations were monozygotic 0.42 and dizygotic 0.06. Both the results of the polychoric correlation and the ACE model indicate strong, although not perfect, heritability for TG.

Green (2000) noted from his clinical practice that he had found three sets of identical transgender twins and suggested genetic involvement, but he did not have enough data to perform statistical analysis.

The Knafo study (Knafo, Iervolino, & Plomin, 2005) used contemporaneous parental ratings of twin gender behavior ratings in the UK Twins Early Development Study (TEDS). They used a model similar to the SEM model that produced loadings on genetic and shared environment. The MTF loading at .26 indicated positive heritability and the FTM loading at .65 indicated strong heritability.

Table 5.2. Studies of heritability of transgenderism. FTM = female to male; GID = gender identity disorder; MTF = male to female; TG = transgenderism.

Year	Author	Type	Children/Teen/Adult	MZ/DZ	TS/TG	MTF/FTM	Number Twin Pairs	Genetic Variance Accounted for	95% Genetic Confidence Interval	% of TS/TG
2000	Bailey et al.	Retrospective survey	Behavior and GID self-ratings	MZ	TG	MTF	312	0.54	.45-.65	N/A
2000	Bailey et al.	Retrospective survey	Behavior and GID self-ratings	MZ	TG	FTM	668	0.42	.31-.49	N/A
2000	Green	Clinical encounter	Adult GID	MZ	TG	MTF/FTM	3	N/A	N/A	N/A
2000	Knafo et al.	Survey 3/4	Parental gender behavior ratings	MZ	TG	MTF	1362	0.26	N/A	N/A
2000	Knafo et al.	Survey 3/4	Gender role behavior ratings	MZ	TG	FTM	1427	0.65	N/A	N/A
2002	Coolidge, et al.	Survey 4/17 years	Parental ratings child GID DSM-IV	MZ	TG	MTF/FTM	96	0.62	N/A	N/A
2006	van Beijseveldt et al.	Survey 7/10 years	Parental behavioral ratings	MZ	TG	MTF/FTM	14000	0.70	N/A	N/A
2010	Heylens et al.	Review clinical	Child GID diagnosis	MZ	TG	MTF/FTM	23	0.00	0	39

Coolidge, Thede, and Young (2002) recruited the parents of twins through advertisement to provide behavioral ratings of their children on a rating scale derived from the items in the gender identity disorder diagnosis of the fourth edition of the *Diagnostic and Statistical Manual of Mental Disorders*. They used the SEM statistical analysis and after preliminary analysis the C factor was dropped because it did not account for much variance. Table 5.1 reveals that there was a strong heritability based on the A scale statistic of 0.62 for the AE model across both MTF and FTM gender nonconformity.

The van Beijsterveldt study (van Beijsterveldt, Hudziak, & Boomsma, 2006) involved mothers' ratings of gender nonconforming behavior at 7 and 10 years. It included monozygotic, dizygotic, and opposite-sex twins from the Netherlands Twin Registry. The SEM model indicated strong heritability for combined MTF and FTM in both age groups at 0.77 and 0.71. MTF and FTM statistics were not reported separately.

The last study was by Heylens et al. (2012), who conducted a literature review to find cases of twins in which one was transgender and found that overall 39% both were TG.

With regard to the heritability survey results shown in Table 5.2, not many of the overtly transgender children will continue to be overtly transgender in adulthood. Adult outcomes are discussed in Chapter 9.

Studies of heritability generally provide strong support for the idea that TSTG is biological in origin and that DNA genetics are a causal factor in TSTG. The correlations are strong when compared with our rules of thumb for the transgender population that are 1% for MTF and .5% for FTM although no formal statistical meta-analysis is possible because of the variations in experimental design. However, epigenetic mechanisms may be involved (as discussed in Chapter 6) because there is statistical "room" for other factors to explain the rest of the variance. The usual next step in establishing a genetic causal factor is to find markers on the DNA molecule that indicate possible genes involved in DNA expression of a trait. The next section describes the results of the search for such markers.

5.3 MARKERS FOR TSTG

Markers are features of DNA that discriminate between traits—in this case, TSTG and non-TSTG. The search for DNA markers for TSTG has been impeded because resources have not yet permitted a full DNA scan. But DNA scans have been completed for other phenomena, such as homosexuality and breast cancer. The experimental design for such investigations involves careful selection of a transsexual group and a control group that should be a matched sample. Alternative designs involve a more brute-force approach by getting large populations of TSTG and control subjects.

Because the resources for a full DNA scan were unavailable, previous investigators have had to guess where to look in the DNA molecule for such markers.

Driven by the hypothesis that TSTG is caused by the presence of low or high prenatal sex hormone levels, the initial investigations were concerned with sex hormone receptor genes and associated genes. This hypothesis turns out to be faulty and is evaluated in the next chapter. The other gene that was hypothesized might be involved with FTM TSTG is in the area of DNA, which is believed to regulate hormonal activity.

As noted earlier, pursuit of full DNA genome scans (and full epigenome scans) is now much less expensive in terms of time and money and is thus now within reach. Epigenome scans are scans that look for chemicals outside of DNA itself that influence DNA expression—for example, by inactivating a gene. Such scans are important to establish DNA heritability but also because many phenomena involve multiple DNA markers.

Table 5.3 shows DNA marker studies for TSTG starting with two studies looking for chromosome anomalies. The Turan et al. (2000) research paper only involved one FTM transsexual who had an extra X chromosome. For that reason, this study is probably not definitive. Many clinics around the world examine chromosomes as part of their regular intake procedure for transsexualism. If an extra X chromosome was a causal factor in transsexualism, one might expect many more research reports on this issue. The Hengstschläger et al. (2003) study did a more detailed chromosome analysis and found two areas for investigation in future studies involving full DNA scans. One was a translocation of a gene pattern, and the other involved increased gene micro deletions on the Y chromosome.

The Henningsson et al. (2005) study looked for TSTG markers by comparing Swedish transsexuals with controls. They did not have the resources to look through the entire DNA genome but guessed that markers might be found on DNA sites involved in hormone receptors (androgen or AR; estrogen or E beta) and aromatase production CYP19 located at 15q21.1. Aromatase is of interest because it is the enzyme that converts testosterone into estradiol in the brain to induce prenatal masculinization (McCarthy, 2008). It is true, but counterintuitive, that estrogen, normally associated with females, actually performs the masculinization role for sexual reflex circuits in the hypothalamus and other places in the brain. Estrogens do not cross into the brain because of active defensive mechanisms, but testosterone does cross and is converted to estradiol by the aromatase enzyme. Subjects were transsexuals from Sweden recruited by three clinics from a national registry.

Henningsson et al. (2005) found that the MTF transsexual AR gene pattern had longer allele repeat lengths than controls. They also determined that in transsexual subjects who had short AR repeat lengths, both the estrogen receptors and aromatase production genes had longer repeat lengths.

Table 5.3. Genetic markers for transsexualism and transgenderism. FTM = female to male; MTF = male to female; SNP = single nucleotide polymorphism.

Year	Author	MTF/FTM	TS/TG	Subjects	Karotype	Type	Location	Result
2000	Turan et al.	FTM	TS	1	47,XXX	Extra X	X	Extra X
2003	Hengstschlager et al.	MTF	TS	30	46,XY	Translocation	46,XY,t(6;17)	1 of 30 Positive for Translocation
2003	Hengstschlager et al.	MTF	TS	31	46,XY	Y microdeletion	Y	Positive Y microdeletions
2005	Henningsson et al.	MTF	TS	29	46,XY	Androgen receptor genes	Sex Xq11-12	Positive
2005	Henningsson et al.	MTF	TS	29	46,XX	Estrogen receptor *Beta* CA	Somatic 14q21-q22	Positive with short AR repeat lengths
2005	Henningsson et al.	MTF	TS	29	46,XX	Aromatase gene CYP19 TTTA	Somatic 15q21.1	Positive with short AR repeat lengths
2009	Hare et al.	MTF	TS	112	46,XY	X androgen receptor	Sex Xq11-12	Positive for longer repeat lengths
2009	Hare et al.	MTF	TS	112	46,XY	Estrogen receptor *Beta* CA	Somatic 14q21-q22	Negative
2009	Hare et al.	MTF	TS	112	46,XY	Aromatase gene CYP19 TTTA	Somatic 15q21.1	Negative

2008	Bentz et al.	FTM	TS	49	46,XX	CYP17 -34 T>C SNP allele frequencies	Somatic 15q21	Positive
2008	Bentz et al.	MTF	TS	102	46,XY	CYP17 -34 T>C SNP allele frequencies	Somatic 15q21	Negative
2009	Ujike et al.	MTF/ FTM	TS	74/168	46,XY; 46,XX	Androgen receptor genes	Sex Xq11-12	Negative
2009	Ujike et al.	MTF/ FTM	TS	74/168	46,XY	Estrogen receptor genes	Somatic 11q13	Negative
2009	Ujike et al.	MTF/ FTM	TS	74/168	46,XY	Estrogen receptor *Beta* CA	Somatic 14q21-q22	Negative
2009	Ujike et al.	MTF/ FTM	TS	74/168	46,XY	Aromatase gene CYP19 TTTA	Somatic 15q21.1	Negative
2009	Ujike et al.	MTF/ FTM	TS	74/168	46,XY	PGR 11q22 polymorphisms	PGR 11q22	Negative

The Hare et al. (2009) study essentially replicated the results of the Henningsson study and employed Australian and United States transsexuals. It was conducted at Monash University and the University of California at Los Angeles. Blood samples were taken, and repeat patterns of genes (alleles) were examined for length. The average repeat length of androgen receptor gene was longer and statistically significantly different from controls. No such effects were found for the estrogen receptor or aromatase-creation alleles.

Bentz et al. (2008) studied Austrian and German FTM transsexuals looking for differences in the CYP17 area of DNA, which contains a site that is associated with elevated levels of testosterone, estradiol, and progesterone. This is because it is believed that the CYP17 area expresses enzymes that catalyze from cholesterol derivative chemicals into these sex hormones. Bentz found that FTM had the same allele pattern in this region as males but not control females, making it a candidate gene for FTM transsexualism.

The Ujike et al. (2009) study was an attempt to replicate and enlarge on the Henningsson et al. (2005) results and was contemporaneous with the Hare et al. (2009) research. Subjects were Japanese transsexuals and age-matched controls. They enlarged the number of investigated DNA sites for the androgen receptor and added an additional estrogen receptor site. As before, they investigated the CYP17 aromatase site. They also looked at the developed progesterone receptors. They found no differences between transsexuals and controls for any of the gene sites they investigated, which they attribute to using Asian as opposed to Caucasian subjects. This negative result is explainable by the fact that country and genetic origin differences have been observed in AR allele repeats (Ackerman et al., 2012; Rajender, Singh, & Kumarasamy, 2007).

The differences that were observed in the repeat 2 of the AR gene for MTF transsexuals should be considered in the context of what is known about the AR gene and this section in particular. Because medical research focuses on disease states, studies have been funded to study what diseases correlate with allele variations in the AR gene. Many studies have been conducted, and, in fact, there is actually a large online database (Gottlieb, 2014). However, there are only a few phenomena that consistently correlate with AR allele variations: androgen insensitivity syndrome, breast cancer, prostate cancer, male infertility, and now MTF TSTG (Bentz et al., 2008; Hare et al., 2009; Henningsson et al., 2005; Rajender, Gupta, Chakravarty, Singh, & Thangaraj 2006; Rajender, Singh, & Thangarai, 2006).

AIS is of particular interest to the study of the phenomena of TSTG. As noted earlier, AIS is a difference in sexual development in which the body does not respond to androgens during development and is associated with mutations of the AR receptor gene. AIS occurs in approximately 1 of 20,400 live births (Bangsboll, Qvist, Lebech, & Lewinsky, 1992). AIS can be complete (CAIS) or partial (PAIS). CAIS is somewhat less likely than PAIS. AIS does not affect 46,XX to any great extent, but it does affect 46,XY. In males, AIS results in natal female sex organ characteristics even though the person may have 46,XY chromosomes that normally result in male sex characteristics.

Mutations of the AR gene are associated with cases of AIS including mutations of the AR receptor gene including the CAG-repeat section, but it may also involve the other seven sections of the gene. Evidence was presented earlier that a mutation of the AR CAG-repeat section is associated with a feminine gender predisposition that brings on MTF TSTG.

It is interesting that 46,XY AIS people do not exhibit large increases in masculine behavior or desire for masculine transition that one would expect if gender predisposition was determined by non-AR genes. One would expect that 46,XY people with AIS would find the masculine gender behavior category to be more congruent. However, masculine behavior and male body change is rare in people with AIS (Mazur, 2005). People with CAIS appear to be satisfied with their assigned gender behavior category (Wisniewski et al., 2000). In a review of the literature Mazur (2005), found no cases of TS genital plastic surgery (GPS) associated with 46,XY CAIS and nine cases associated with PAIS. Subsequently, one CAIS patient has been reported who underwent TS GPS (Kulshrestha et al., 2009; T'Sjoen et al., 2011) and only one additional PAIS patient who completed TS GPS (Gooren & Cohen-Kettenis, 1991).

In the case of AIS, it appears that AR mutations including CAG-repeat mutations create a feminine gender predisposition as well as preventing the effects of androgens on development. Feminine gender predisposition would be congruent with a feminine gender behavior category to which most 46,XY are assigned and thus the feminine gender behavior would be congruent for 46,XY AIS people. The masculine gender behavior category and male body change would be incongruent for them.

This evidence lends further support to the idea that understanding AR receptor gene mutations is important for understanding the biological basis for TSTG. However, for TSTG we currently have information only on the CAG-repeat section of the AR gene because of limited resources for TSTG research. This is juxtaposed to the huge resources devoted to the study of the AR gene in disease states. TSTG science in this area would greatly benefit from additional AR gene research.

Research on the FTM marker identified earlier is important both to an understanding of TSTG causation and also to FTM health. The CYP17 -34 T>C marker for FTM, in the CYP17 gene has been investigated as a possible contributor to polycystic ovary syndrome (PCOS), which occurs somewhat more frequently in FTM than controls (Mueller et al., 2008; Pache et al., 1991). PCOS is associated with the ovaries releasing high levels of androgens that may result in the growth of ovarian cysts and other negative effects. Several genes have been suspected of mediating PCOS, and results to date are inconsistent because of small sample size and selection (Diamanti-Kandarakis,

Kandarakis, & Legro, 2006; Fauser et al., 2011). Increased PCOS susceptibility in FTM may be due to higher baseline androgen levels in FTM even for those who have not started HT, rather than a direct relationship with DNA genetics (Mueller et al., 2008; Pache et al., 1991). FTM transsexuals may be more at risk for PCOS because they have higher initial levels of androgens combined with the additional androgens they take as part of HT (see Section 13.2.2.2.2).

The results of marker studies indicate the existence of DNA markers which are likely to be involved in TSTG. There are different markers for MTF TSTG and FTM TSTG. Since several genes control most traits, the finding of TSTG markers consists of an "existence proof" and not the final identification of the genes involved in TSTG.

5.4 FTM GENETIC BIOMETRICS

There are several biometric studies that support genetic involvement in FTM TSTG. The first was a study of tooth diameter (Antoszewski, Kruk-Jeromin, & Malinowski, 1998; Antoszewski, Zadzinska, & Foczpanski, 2009) that included FTM transsexuals, non-FTM females, and non-TSTG males. Tooth diameters are believed by the authors to be determined by genetics and differ between the sexes. Whether the FTM transsexuals were on hormone therapy was not reported. The FTM transsexual diameters were intermediate between male and female diameters for six particular teeth types.

The second biometric study (Scitek, Fijalkowska, Zadinska, & Antoszewski, 2012) was of characteristics of pelvic bones for FTM and control male and female patients who reported to the clinic complaining of pelvic pain. Pelvic characteristics are believed by the authors to be determined by genetics and differ between males and females. FTM in the study were on HT. Discriminant analysis indicated differences in the pelvis for FTM TS that was shifted toward the control males. The study by Scitek, Fijalkowska, Zadinska, and Antoszewski (2012) also included a literature review that indicated that FTM have been found to be intermediate between males and females in terms of other biometrics including waist-to-hip ratio, body-weight to body-height ratio, chest-circumference to body-height ratio, and other metrics.

These studies confirm genetic differences exist between FTM transsexuals and non-FTM females.

5.5 GENETICS OF 2D:4D FINGER LENGTH RATIO

The 2D:4D ratio is the ratio between the length of the second finger and the length of the fourth finger and it has been found to correlate with TSTG. The 2D:4D ratio is known from other research to have a strong genetic basis.

Results show that 2D:4D ratio correlates with TSTG. The ratio is higher in MTF and lower in FTM transsexuals in the opposite natal sex range.

The first study of 2D:4D in transsexuals was conducted by Schneider, Pickel, and Stalla (2005), who found that the 2D:4D ratio of the right hand was higher in MTF but not in FTM transsexuals. Kraemer et al. (2009) found that the 2D:4D ratios of the right hand for both MTF and FTM transsexuals were higher than natal sex controls. MTF ratios were in the female range. In children and adult transgender people, Wallien, Zucker, Steensma, and Cohen-Kettenis (2008) found that adult transgender women had lower mean ratio than natal female sex controls. However, Wallien, Zucker, Steensma, and Cohen-Kettenis (2008) did not find any significant difference for MTF transgender people or for transgender FTM children. Hisause, Sasaki, Tsukamoto, and Horie (2012) found that the 2D:4D ratio for FTM was lower (toward the male range) than for natal female controls.

There is evidence for a genetic causal factor for 2D:4D ratio. Paul, Kato, Cherkas, Andrew, and Spector (2006) found in a twin study that the loading for the 2D:4D ratio was 66%, indicating that 2D:4D heritability was high. When compared with the high standard of body height heritability of 60% to 80%, this represents a strong correlation. Gobrogge, Breedlove, and Klump (2008) obtained similar results and found that the correlation was higher for monozygotic than for dizygotic twins. Hiraishi, Saski, Shikishima, and Ando (2012) obtained similar results as the preceding two studies for a twin sample from Japan except that the finding of heritability was found for both left and right hands.

It is believed that finger length is controlled by the 39 genes that are found on chromosomes 2, 7, 12, and 17 (Goodman & Scambler, 2001; Sheth et al., 2012). Zhang (Zhang et al., 2013) found that the 2D:4D ratio did not correlate with repeats on the AR gene. Voracek (2008) found that 2D:4D ratio varied with blood type, indicating the potential that known genes that determine blood type might also govern 2D:4D ratio.

Supporting a genetic causal factor for 2D:4D is the fact that this ratio varies with different populations around the world. Loehlin, McFadden, Medland, and Martin (2006) found differences among populations in the United States, Britain, and Australia. The authors found that the results indicated a primary gene pool effect.

These studies confirm that the genetic mechanism of the 2D:4D ratio is strong and well characterized by human and animal studies, which means that epigenetic mechanisms play a small role. This provides further support for the genetics as a causal factor in TSTG.

The correlation between TSTG and 2D:4D ratio is often cited as evidence for the prenatal testosterone epigenetic theory of transsexual causation (as discussed in Chapter 6), but the evidence presented above indicates that there is hardly any statistical room for a contribution by an epigenetic causal factor to 2D:4D ratios.

5.6 GENETIC MECHANISMS

The evidence that supports a DNA genetic causal factor for TSTG does not tell us what mechanisms are involved at the next lowest level of explanation, but there are at least three possible purely genetic mechanism categories for TSTG.

There are three potential well-understood DNA genetic mechanism categories for TSTG. (1) **Germline DNA** passed on from parents' DNA might provide a mechanism. There may be genetic pressure to pass on diverse genes that are useful to the clan, family, or tribe, or genetic drift may be involved. (2) Another potential mechanism involves a DNA **de novo mutation** during conception, a mutation that neither parent possesses. (3) More recently, in regard to another potential mechanism, it has been found that some people are **mosaics**, meaning that they have more than one type of DNA in their bodies. It has been discovered that the brain is a haven for all types of DNA, and one possible mechanism for genetic TSTG is that cells with foreign DNA may create a gender behavior predisposition in the brain that is independent of DNA in the rest of the body.

5.6.1 Germline Mechanisms

At conception, germline DNA from parents might provide the basis for a purely genetic mechanism. Parental DNA has been influenced by selective pressures from the moment the human species started. There may have been genetic pressures to pass on diverse genes that are useful to the clan, family, or tribe. Examples can be found in the Native American tribes in which it was an advantage to have two-spirit people who had the flexibility to alternately act as warriors or weavers or engage in child rearing in the harsh environment in which they lived.

5.6.2 De Novo Mutations

Another potential mechanism involves a DNA de novo mutation. The mutation can occur in the female egg or male sperm after release but before or just at conception. In this case, the DNA mutation is not due to either of the parents' DNA. There are many phenomena, including diseases, that result from de novo mutations.

5.6.3 Multiple DNA

More recently, potential mechanisms have been discovered indicating that many people have more than one type of DNA in their bodies, a phenomenon known as **mosaicism**. Some mosaicism involves only a few genes but some involves whole sets of genes. These discoveries were largely due to the wide-spread use of genetic testing for establishing paternity/maternity and for processing evidence from crime scenes. Mosaicism is counterintuitive because in most cases, hosts attack cells with foreign DNA. This is why medical personnel take great care to find DNA matches to avoid tissue rejection in bone marrow transplants and organ transplantations. However, it turns out that under some circumstances, people can have multiple DNA in their bodies without rejection. In particular, it appears as though the brain is a safe haven for cells with all kinds of DNA.

Mosaicism involves formation of multiple DNA species at conception or shortly thereafter. Mosaicism can occur when differences in DNA are formed due to mistakes in cell copying, particularly just after conception.

Several recent studies have considered mosaicism, but none have tested the hypothesis that mosaicism may be involved in TSTG. Chan et al. (2012) found that cells and genetic material transfered from the fetus to the mother could persist in the brain and body creating mosaicism. The exchange presumably goes in both directions between fetus and mother. Cogle et al. (2004) found genetic material from a bone marrow transplant involving a male donor and a female recipient. Later cells were found in the brain with a Y chromosome, indicating that some of the donor cells migrated and flourished in the brain of the female. Reed, Lee, Norris, Utter, & Busch (2007) also reported chimerism after blood transfusions. It is widely known in animal husbandry that genetic material can be transferred between opposite-sex twin calves in utero but Bogdanova et al. (2010) found mosaicism in a female human resulting from transfer of genetic material from a human male twin.

Humans are all true mosaics because they have many different DNA sequences in cells of the brain, all of which seem to be tolerated. Coufal (2009) compared the human genes in brain and body and found that the brain was significantly mosaicked by "jumping genes" that copy themselves to other parts of the genome compared with the body cells. He found that some brain samples had more than 100 copies of these jumping genes. In a more recent study, McConnell et al. (2013) found that the copy numbers of brain neurons varied widely. Copy number reflects the number of mutations in the genome. The results indicated mosaicking is common in the brain.

A particularly interesting type of mosaicism is called **tetragametic chimerism**, which occurs when two fertilized eggs merge within a few days after conception. At this point in development, the eggs do not reject the presence of foreign cells. A chimera is a type of mosaic that has two sets of DNA. A case study of chimerism was provided by Neng (2002), and a British documentary film of this and another case is available (BBC Channel Five, 2006). In these cases, both eggs were 46,XX but tetragametic chimerism is of particular interest if one of the eggs is 46,XX and the other 46,XY. Such people have DNA of both sexes. The obvious question is what DNA is in their brain, and what is their gender predisposition? There are only few known people who are tetragametic chimera, but there is an autobiography of one who was MTF (Alden, 2013). We have not been able to correlate the presence of multiple DNA species with TSTG, but this should be possible in the future. It also may allow us to determine which somatic and sex chromosomes and genes are involved in TSTG.

In essence, everyone is a mosaic when it comes to the brain including transsexuals and transgender people. The brain also contains DNA species that have mutated from the original DNA and many genes have moved location (McConnell et al., 2013). The possibility exists that the DNA in some cells may create a gender behavior predisposition in the brain that is independent of DNA in the rest of the body. These studies also beg the questions as to whether gender behavior predisposition is linked to DNA sex traits at all and could TSTG be due to the DNA in maternal or sibling cells that have migrated into the fetus during pregnancy.

5.7 CONSANGINITY

Consanginity refers to having offspring with a close blood relative. Such inbreeding frequently results in undesirable genetic defects. Most cultures and religions ban marriages between cousins or close relatives for this reason. Historically, however, many royal families have conducted inbreeding with their cousins or even their siblings to consolidate power. Walinder and Thuwe (1977) investigated the possibility of consanguinity in transsexuals and found that none of the 61 transsexuals he examined in his study reported such relationships with their cousins or close relatives.

5.8 SUMMARY

On the basis of the evidence contained in this chapter, six conclusions should be drawn. First, there is substantial evidence indicating that TSTG is heritable due to DNA genetic effects based on twin and family studies of heritability. The second conclusion is that there are DNA genetic markers for TSTG that confirm this DNA genetic causal factor. The third conclusion is that genetic heritability is not the whole story. If one uses body height as a reference for the limit of heritability, there is still statistical room for other causal factors to explain the remaining statistical variance. Statistics show that heritability is moderate to strong. In the next chapter, we examine the evidence for an epigenetic causal factor to explain the remaining variance. In Chapter 7 we explore a two-factor theory of TSTG causation.

The fourth conclusion is that there is genetics science support for the idea that TSTG is biological in nature. The fifth conclusion is that AIS is associated with the same AR gene mutation that causes feminine gender predisposition. It appears that this feminine gender predisposition is responsible for MTF TSTG and the high frequency of 46,XY AIS congruity with a feminine gender behavior category. The sixth conclusion is that the 2D:4D finger ratio correlates with TSTG and it appears that it varies primarily with a genetic factor.

REFERENCES

Ackerman, C., Lowe, L. P., Lee, H., Hayes, M. G., Dyer, A. R., Metzger, B. E., . . . Urbanek, M.; Hapo Study Cooperative Research Group. (2012). Ethnic variation in allele distribution of the androgen receptor (CAG)n repeat. *Journal of Andrology, 33*, 210–215.

Alden, J. (2013). *A season for April, Part I: summer storms.* Kindle. Amazon Digital Services. Available at http://www.amazon.com/Season-April-Part -Summer-Storms-ebook/dp/B00DT4LHL0.

Antoszewski, B., Kruk-Jeromin, J., & Malinowski, A. (1998). Body structure of female-to-male transsexuals. *Acta Chirurgica Plastica, 40*, 54–58.

Antoszewski, B., Zadzinska, E., & Foczpanski, J. (2009). The metric features of teeth in female-to-male transsexuals. *Archives of Sexual* Behavior, *38*, 351–358.

Bailey, J., Dunne, M., & Martin, N. (2000). Genetic and environmental influences on sexual orientation and its correlates in an Australian twin sample. *Journal of Personality and Social Psychology, 78*, 524–536.

Bailey, J., & Zucker, K. (1995, January). Childhood sex-typed behavior and sexual orientation: A conceptual analysis and quantitative review. *Developmental Psychology, 31*, 43–55.

Bangsboll, S., Qvist, I., Lebech, P., & Lewinsky, M. (1992). Testicular feminization syndrome and associated gonadal tumors in Denmark. *Acta Obstetrica Gynecologica Scandinavica, 71*, 63–66.

BBC Channel Five. (2006, May 26). *The twin inside me* [episode 5 of *Extraordinary People*]. (Released in the United States as *I am my own twin*.) Retrieved April 30, 2014, from http://web.archive.org/web/20060526105634/ http://www.five.tv/programmes/extraordinarypeople/twininside.

Bentz, E., Hefler, L. A., Kaufmann, U., Huber, J. C., Kolbus, A., & Tempfer, C. B. (2008). A polymorphism of the CYP17 gene related to sex steroid metabolism is associated with female-to-male but not male-to-female transsexualism. *Fertility and Sterility, 90*, 57–59.

Bogdanova, N., Siebers, U., Kelsch, R., Markoff, A., Röpke, A., Exeler, R., . . . Wieacker, P. (2010, May). Blood chimerism in a girl with Down syndrome and possible freemartin effect leading to aplasia of the Mullerian derivatives. *Human Reproduction, 25*, 1339–1343.

Bruder, C., Piotrowski, A., Gijsbers, A. A., Andersson, R., Erickson, S., Diaz de Ståhl, T., . . . Dumanski, J. P. (2008). Phenotypically concordant and discordant monozygotic twins display different DNA copy-number-variation profiles. *American Journal of Human Genetics, 82,* 763–771.

Chan, W. F. N., Gurnot, C., Montine, T. J., Sonnen, J. A., Guthrie, K. A., & Nelson, J. L. (2012). Male microchimerism in the human female brain. *PLoS ONE, 7,* e45592.

Chao-Qiang, L. (2006, December 11). How much of human height is genetic and how much is due to nutrition? *Scientific American.* Retrieved April 16, 2014, from http://www.scientificamerican.com/article/how-much-of -human-height.

Clancy, S. (2008). RNA functions. *Nature Education, 1*(1), 102.

Cogle, C., Yachnis, A. T., Laywell, E. D., Zander, D. S., Wingard, J. R., Steindler, D. A., & Scott, E. W. (2004, May). Bone marrow transdifferentiation in brain after transplantation: A retrospective study. *Lancet, 363,* 1432–1437.

Coolidge, F., Thede, L., & Young, S. (2002). The heritability of gender identity disorder in a child and adolescent twin sample. *Behavior Genetics, 32,* 251–257.

Coufal, N. (2009). L1 retrotransposition in human neural progenitor cells. *Nature, 460,* 1127–1131.

Diamanti-Kandarakis, E., Kandarakis, H., & Legro, R. (2006). The role of genes and environment in the etiology of PCOS. *Endocrine, 30,* 19–26.

Diamond, M. (2013). Transsexuality among twins: Identity concordance, transition, rearing and orientation. *International Journal of Transgenderism, 14,* 24–38.

Fauser, B., Diedrich, K., Bouchard, P., Domínguez, F., Matzuk, M., Franks, S., . . . Howles, C. M. (2011). Contemporary genetic technologies and female reproduction. *Human Reproduction Update, 17,* 829–847.

Gobrogge, K., Breedlove, S., & Klump, K. (2008). Genetic and environmental influences on 2D:4D finger length ratios: A study of monozygotic and dizygotic male and female twins. *Archives of Sexual Behavior, 37,* 112–118.

Gómez-Gil, E., Esteva, I., Almaraz, M. C., Pasaro, E., Segovia, S., & Guillamon, A. (2010). Familiality of gender identity disorder in non-twin siblings. *Archives of Sexual Behavior, 39,* 546–552.

Goodman, F., & Scambler, P. (2001). Human HOX gene mutations. *Clinical Genetics, 59,* 1–11.

Gooren, L., & Cohen-Kettenis, P. (1991, October). Development of male gender identity/role and a sexual orientation towards women in a 46,XY subject with an incomplete form of the androgen insensitivity syndrome. *Archives of Sexual Behavior, 20,* 459–470.

Gordon, L., Joo, J. E., Powell, J. E., Ollikainen, M., Novakovic, B., Li, X., Andronikos, R., . . . Saffrey, R. (2012). Neonatal DNA methylation profile in human twins is specified by a complex interplay between intrauterine environmental and genetic factors, subject to tissue-specific influence. *Genome Research, 22,* 1395–1406.

Gottlieb, B. (2014). The androgen receptor gene mutation database. McGill University. Retrieved April 16, 2014, from http://androgendb.mcgill.ca.

Green, R. (1979, January). Childhood cross-gender behavior and subsequent sexual preference. *American Journal of Psychiatry, 136,* 106–108.

Green, R. (2000). Family co-occurrence of "gender dysphoria": Ten sibling or parent–child pairs. *Archives of Sexual Behavior, 29,* 499–507.

Hare, L., Bernard, P., Sánchez, F. J., Baird, P. N., Vilain, E., Kennedy, T., & Harley, V. R. (2009). Androgen receptor repeat length polymorphism associated with male-to-female transsexualism. *Biological Psychiatry, 65,* 93–96.

Hengstschläger, M., von Trostenburg, M., Repa, C., Marton, E., Huber, J. C., & Bernaschek, G. (2003). Sex chromosome aberrations and transsexualism. *Fertility and Sterility, 79,* 639–640.

Henningsson, S., Westberg, L., Nilsson, S., Lundstrom, B., Ekseliusd, L., & Bodlunde, O. (2005). Sex steroid-related genes and male-to-female transsexualism. *Psychoneuroendocrinology, 30,* 657–664.

Hepp, U., Milos, G., & Braun-Scharm, H. (2003, February). Gender identity disorder and anorexia nervosa in male monozygotic twins. *International Journal of Eating Disorders, 35,* 239–243.

Heylens, G., De Cuypere, G., Zucker, K. J., Schelfaut, C., Elaut, E., Vanden Bossche, H., . . . & T'Sjoen, G. (2012, March). Gender identity disorder in twins: A review of the case report literature. *Journal of Sexual Medicine, 9,* 751–757.

Hiraishi, K., Saski, S., Shikishima, C., & Ando, J. (2012, June). The second to fourth digit ratio (2D:4D) in a Japanese twin sample: Heritability, prenatal hormone transfer, and association with sexual orientation. *Archives of Sexual Behavior, 41,* 711–724.

Hisause, S., Sasaki, S., Tsukamoto, T., & Horie, S. (2012). The relationship between second-to-fourth digit ratio and female gender identity. *Journal of Sexual Medicine, 9,* 2903–2910.

Hyde, C., & Kenna, J. (1977, October). A male MZ twin pair, concordant for transsexualism, discordant for schizophrenia. *Acta Psychiatrica Scandinavica, 56,* 265–275.

Joyce, P., & Ding, L. (1985, June). Transsexual sisters. *Australia and New Zealand Journal of Psychiatry, 19,* 188–189.

Knafo, A., Iervolino, A., & Plomin, R. (2005). Masculine girls and feminine boys: Genetic and environmental contributions to atypical gender development in early childhood. *Journal of Personal and Social Psychology, 88,* 400–412.

Knoblauch, H., Busjahn, A., & Wegener, B. (2007). Monozygotic twins concordant for female-to-male transsexualism: A case report. *Archives of Sexual Behavior, 36,* 135–137.

Kraemer, B., Noll, T., Delsignore, A., Milos, G., Schnyder, U., & Hepp, U. (2009). Finger length ratio (2D:4D) in adults with gender identity disorder. *Archives of Sexual Behavior, 38,* 359–363.

Kulshrestha, B., Philibert, P., Eunice, M., Khandelwal, S. K., Mehta, M., Audran, F., . . . Ammini, A. C. (2009, December). Apparent male gender identity in a patient with complete androgen insensitivity syndrome. *Archives of Sexual Behavior, 38,* 873–875.

Liu, F., van Duijn, K., Vingerling, J. R., Hofman, A., Uitterlinden, A. G., Janssens, A. C., & Kayser, M. (2009, March 10). Eye color and the prediction of complex phenotypes from genotypes. *Current Biology, 19,* R192–R193.

Loehlin, J., McFadden, D., Medland, S., & Martin, N. (2006). Population differences in finger-length ratios: Ethnicity or latitude? *Archives of Sexual Behavior, 35,* 739–742.

Mazur, T. (2005, August). Gender dysphoria and gender change in androgen insensitivity or micropenis. *Archives of Sexual Behavior, 34,* 411–421.

McCarthy, M. (2008). Estradiol and the developing brain. *Physiology Review, 88,* 91–124.

McConnell, M., Lindberg, M. R., Brennarnd, K. J., Piper, J. C., Voet, T., Cowling-Zitron, C., . . . Gage, F. H. (2013). Mosaic copy number variation in human neurons. *Science, 342,* 632–637.

Mueller, A., Gooren, L., Naton-Schotz, S., Cupisti, S., Beckman, M., & Dittrich, R. (2008). Prevalence of polycystic ovary syndrome and hyperandrogenemia in female-to-male transsexuals. *Journal of Clinical Endocrinology and Metabolism, 93,* 1408–1411.

Neng, et al. (2002). Disputed maternity leading to identification of tetragametic chimerism. *New England Journal of Medicine, 346,* 1545-1552.

Pache, T., Chadha, S., Gooren, L. J., Hop, W. C., Jaarsma, K. W., Dommerholt, H. B., & Fauser, B. C. (1991, November). Ovarian morphology in long-term androgen-treated female to male transsexuals. A human model for the study of polycystic ovarian syndrome? *Histopathology, 19,* 445–452.

Paul, S., Kato, B., Cherkas, L., Andrew, T., & Spector, T. (2006, April). Heritability of the second to fourth digit ratio (2d:4d): A twin study. *Twin Research and Human Genetics, 9,* 215–219.

Rajender, S., Gupta, N., Chakravarty, B., Singh, L., & Thangaraj, K. (2008). Androgen insensitivity syndrome: Do trinucleotide repeats in androgen receptor gene have any role? *Asian Journal of Andrology, 10,* 616–624.

Rajender, S., Singh, L., & Kumarasamy, T. (2007). Phenotypic heterogeneity of mutations in androgen receptor gene. *Asian Journal of Andrology, 29,* 147–179.

Reed, W., Lee, T., Norris, P., Utter, G., & Busch, M. (2007). Transfusion-associated microchimerism: A new complication of blood transfusions in severely injured patients. *Seminars in Hematology, 44,* 24–31.

Sabalis, R., Frances, A., Appenzeller, S., & Mosely, W. (1974, August). The three sisters: Transsexual male siblings. *American Journal of Psychiatry, 131*, 907–909.

Sadeghi, M., & Fakhrai, A. (2002). Transsexualism in female monozygotic twins: A case report. *Behavior Genetics, 32*, 862–864.

Schneider, H., Pickel, J., & Stalla, G. (2005). Typical female 2nd–4th finger length (2D:4D) ratios in male-to-female transsexuals—possible implications for prenatal androgen exposure. *Psychoneuroendocrinology, 31*, 265–269.

Scitek, A., Fijalkowska, M., Zadinska, E., & Antoszewski, B. (2012). Biometric characteristics of the pelvis in female-to-male transsexuals. *Archives of Sexual Behavior, 41*, 1303–1313.

Segal, N. (2006, June). Two monozygotic twin pairs discordant for female-to-male transsexualism. *Archives of Sexual Behavior, 35*, 347–358.

Sheth, R., Marcon, L., Bastida, M. F., Junco, M., Auintana, L., Dahn, R., . . . Ros, M. A. (2012). *Hox* genes regulate digit patterning by controlling the wavelength of a Turing-type mechanism. *Science, 338*, 1476–1480.

T'Sjoen, G., De Cuypere, G., Monstrey, S., Hoebeke, P., Freedman, F. K., Appari, M., . . . Cools, M. (2011). Male gender identity in complete androgen insensitivity syndrome. *Archives of Sexual Behavior, 40*, 635–638.

Turan, M., Eşel, E., Dündar, M., Candemir, Z., Baştürk, M., Sofuoğlu, S., Ozkul, Y., et al. (2000). Female-to-male transsexual with 47, XXX karyotype. *Biological Psychiatry, 48*, 1116–1117.

Ujike, H., Otani, K., Nakatsuka, M., Ishii, K., Sasaki, A., Oishi, T., . . . Kuroda S. (2009). Association study of gender identity disorder and sex-hormone related genes. *Progress in Neuropsychopharmacology and Biological Psychiatry, 33*, 1241–1244.

van Beijsterveldt, C., Hudziak, J., & Boomsma, D. (2006). Genetic and environment influences on cross-gender behavior and relation to behavior problems: A study of Dutch twins at ages 7 and 10. *Archives of Sexual Behavior, 35*, 647–658.

Veale, J., Clarke, D., & Lomax, T. (2010). Biological and psychosocial correlates of adult gender-variant identities: A review. *Personality and Individual Differences, 48*, 351–366.

Vilain, E., & McCabe, E. (1998, October). Mammalian sex determination: From gonads to brain. *Molecular Genetics and Metabolism, 65*, 74–84.

Voracek, M. (2008). Digit ratio (2D:4D), ABO blood type, and the Rhesus factor. *Perceptual and Motor Skills, 107*, 737–746.

Walinder, J., & Thuwe, I. (1977). A study of consanguinity between the parents of transsexuals. *British Journal of Psychiatry, 131*, 73–74.

Wallien, M., Zucker, K., Steensma, T., & Cohen-Kettenis, P. (2008). 2D:4D finger-length ratios in children and adults with gender identity disorder. *Hormones and Behavior, 54*, 450–454.

Westberg, L., Baghaei, F., Rosmond, R., Hellstrand, M., Landén, M., Jansson, M., . . . Eriksson, E. (2001). Polymorphisms of the androgen receptor gene and the estrogen receptor beta gene are associated with androgen levels in women. *Journal of Clinical Endocrinology and Metabolism, 86,* 2562–2568.

Wisniewski, A., Migeon, C. J., Meyer-Bahlburg, H. F., Gearhart, J. P., Berkovitz, G. D., Brown, T. R., & Money, J. (2000, August). Complete androgen insensitivity syndrome: Long-term medical, surgical, and psychosexual outcome. *Journal of Clinical Endocrinology and Metabolism, 85,* 2664–2669.

Zhang, C., Dang, J., Pei, L., Guo, M., Zhu, H., Qu, L., . . . Huo, Z. (2013). Relationship of 2D:4D finger ratio with androgen receptor CAG and GGN repeat polymorphism. *American Journal of Human Biology, 25,* 101–106.

6

Epigenetic Causal Factor in Transsexualism and Transgenderism

6.0 INTRODUCTION

There is positive evidence that epigenetics are a causal factor in transsexualism and transgenderism (TSTG), but at this point it is only suggestive that future research should be conducted. More research needs to be performed to confirm the epigenetic mechanisms that have been supported by initial research. Several epigenetic mechanisms have been hypothesized but not supported by the scientific evidence. Epigenetics is a young science, and an increasing number of hypotheses and mechanisms are available for testing.

Epigenetics is a candidate causal factor in TSTG because of the early realization of TSTG starting at age 4 and because of the lack of evidence for child rearing and parental interaction as causal factors. Therefore only causal factors that can have influence before the realization of transgenderism starting at age 4 are candidate causal factors for TSTG. Chapter 8 presents scientific evidence that refutes child rearing or parental interaction as causal factors.

Epigenetics involves the study of mechanisms that modify DNA or change its expression and thus shape the body (phenotype) of a person and/or behavior. Most of these mechanisms begin at conception, but some actually precede conception. An example of the power of epigenetics is that although identical twins start out with the same DNA at conception, epigenetic mechanisms cause considerable differences in their bodies and brains by the time of birth

(Bruder et al., 2008; Gordon et al., 2012). Epigenetics fits with the timing of the early emergence of TSTG. Epigenetic science provides evidence for a causal factor in TSTG and also confirms that TSTG is a biological phenomenon.

This chapter describes potential epigenetic mechanisms for TSTG; Chapter 7 deals with mechanisms in which the interaction of genetic and/or epigenetic mechanisms is suspected. There are several types of epigenetic mechanisms, but the most pertinent to TSTG are imprinting, prenatal endogenous testosterone, toxic drugs, toxic chemicals, and maternal stress effects.

There is a fuzzy line between mechanisms considered to be genetic and those considered epigenetic. The timeline of parental genetics, conception, and development does not provide a distinct division. Epigenetic mechanisms mainly act after conception, but some epigenetic mechanisms can be passed on from parents. Some phenomena (for example, exposure to toxic chemicals) can result in both genetic mutation and changes in how some genes are expressed. We discuss candidate epigenetic mechanisms for TSTG in this chapter, but multiple actions of epigenetic modification sources confirm that a two-factor theory is necessary, as described in Chapter 7.

Imprinting involves transmission to an offspring of a chemical message that changes gene expression but is not part of the DNA molecule itself. This epigenetic mechanism begins before conception. The best understood example of imprinting involves two related phenomena—Angelman syndrome and Prader-Willi syndrome. They both involve a hereditary defect in chromosome 15 that results in loss of function. The symptoms of Angelman syndrome are severe cognitive impairment, speech impairment, movement difficulties, and often seizures. The symptoms of Prader-Willi are obesity and moderate cognitive impairment. Angelman syndrome involves more severe symptoms. If the defect is passed on by the female parent then the child gets Angelman syndrome. However, if the defect is passed on by the male father, a chemical imprint can also be passed on that silences some of the mutated genes on chromosome 15 and leads to the less severe outcome, Prader-Willi. Silencing or repression means that a chemical binds to one or more genes and inhibits them from expression. If only one gene is involved in imprinting, the silencing is through methylation in which a methyl chemical radical (one carbon atom bonded to three hydrogen atoms) binds to a gene. If multiple genes are silenced, a histone mechanism is involved that binds to multiple genes and inhibits their expression. Histone normally acts as a chemical spool around which DNA winds.

Imprinting is a suspected epigenetic causal mechanism of TSTG because of findings that indicate transsexuals have more maternal aunts than uncles. This may indicate a mechanism that prevents males from coming to term unless they have protective DNA inheritances from one or more parents. Alternatively, having more maternal aunts and uncles could involve an epigenetic mechanism based on immune system chemical messengers or on chemicals that modify DNA expression. To date, however, this research study has not been replicated.

Epigenetic imprinting mechanisms of sibling order and sibling sex ratio were thought to be involved in TSTG but subsequent studies revealed that the effects observed were due to homosexuality, not TSTG. As pointed out in Chapter 3, people can be both TSTG and homosexual. Sibling numbers have also been shown to correlate with homosexuality. On the basis of animal experiments, it has been suggested that TSTG is caused by the level of testosterone in the developing fetus, but this candidate mechanism is refuted by several lines of evidence.

Developmental toxicity can occur during the prenatal period. It involves exposure to chemicals that cause DNA genetic mutations and/or changes in DNA expression. These effects can come from the administration of therapeutic drugs, from exposure to toxic chemicals, and from maternal stress.

It is a common misconception that endogenous fetal hormones, especially testosterone, cause transsexualism. This is the **prenatal testosterone theory of transsexualism**. Although it is true, based on animal research, that exogenous testosterone can alter sexual reflexes, sexual behavior, and aggressive behavior, the evidence indicates that levels of prenatal testosterone are not responsible for TSTG in humans. Research in this area is confined to animal behavior, and animals do not have sophisticated gender behavioral categories like humans. There are five other lines of scientific evidence that can be cited to refute the prenatal testosterone theory of transsexualism. This misconception of prenatal testosterone theory of transsexualism has a long history, going back into the eugenics movements in the early 20th century. The theory was initially suggested that transsexualism could be eliminated by injecting pregnant women with systemic testosterone (MTF) or blockers (FTM). As far as we know, such a human experiment has never been done, but the theory lives on in scientific and popular thought.

6.1 IMPRINTING AND TSTG

Green and Keverne (2000) found that MTF transsexuals had more maternal aunts than uncles given a sample of 417 MTF transsexuals. No such relationship was found in a group of 96 FTM transsexuals. The effect was also not found on the paternal side of MTF or FTM. Green interpreted this finding to mean that the mother of the aunts and uncles had inherited an imprinting chemical on one of her X chromosomes that selectively reduced survival of prenatal males but not females. Only those males who were feminized survived. This imprint continued into the next generation on the maternal side. This study is particularly interesting because of its relatively large subject population, which is rare for studies of transsexualism. However, it has never been replicated or followed up.

Three possible imprinting mechanisms for TSTG have been examined, and initial studies found a positive relationship. However, subsequent studies indicated that the effects were due to homosexuality rather than TSTG.

An initial study indicated that TSTG is associated with an imprinting mechanism that correlates with sibling sex ratio (Green, 2000), but the preponderance of evidence from other studies indicates that homosexuality and not TSTG was responsible for the observed effect. There are imprinting mechanisms that are associated with **sibling sex ratio**, but they seem to be associated with homosexuality, not TSTG. Some studies replicated the Green (2000) findings. The first studies included homosexual transgender people (Blanchard & Sheridan, 1992). These studies were replicated by Blanchard and colleagues (Blanchard, Zucker, Bradley, & Hume, 1995; Blanchard, Zucker, Cohen-Kettenis, Gooren, & Bailey, 1996). Zucker, Blanchard, Kim, Pae, and Lee (2007) obtained a similar result in transgender homosexual boys and in Korean homosexuals. The same was found for transgender adolescents (Schagen et al., 2012). It was also found in this study that FTM transgender adolescents had fewer siblings overall. Additional evidence indicates that sibling sex ratio effects were actually associated with homosexuality, not TSTG. One study found that transgender subjects had more brothers than sisters in a sample of MTF homosexual but not nonhomosexual transgender subjects (Blanchard & Sheridan, 1992). Green (2000) found that homosexual transsexuals but not nonhomosexual transsexuals had higher male/female sex ratios compared with control subjects. Green and Keverne (2000) replicated this with a larger sample size. Gómez-Gil et al. (2010) replicated the Green studies (Green, 2000; Green & Keverne, 2000) but included an FTM transsexual group determined by sexual orientation. This study found higher male sibling sex ratios in MTF and FTM transsexual homosexuals but not in nonhomosexual MTF and FTM groups.

The results for **sibling order** are similar to those for sibling sex ratio except that there is more evidence linking sibling order to homosexuality but not TSTG. Males were more likely to be homosexual if they had older male siblings in the Blanchard and Sheridan (1992) study. Some studies found a male homosexual transsexual sibling order effect but did not include a nonhomosexual control group (Blanchard, Zucker, Bradley, & Hume, 1995; Blanchard, Zucker, Cohen-Kettenis, Gooren, & Bailey, 1996; Schagen et al., 2012; Zucker et al., 1997). The sibling sex ratio studies cited earlier also found a sibling order effect for homosexuality but not TSTG (Green, 2000; Green & Keverne, 2000). Gómez-Gil et al. (2010) observed the effect in male MTF homosexual transsexuals but not female FTM homosexual transsexuals. Gomez-Gil et al. also did not observe the order effect in nonhomosexual MTF and FTM control groups.

Studies of homosexual **sibling births** indicates that sibling birth order is associated with homosexuality. In two large Canadian surveys of male subjects, Bogaert (2003a; 2003b) found that the probability of being homosexual increased with the number of older brothers. Bogaert (2004) also found that the population frequency of male homosexuality varied with the fertility rate of a country. Cantor, Blanchard, Paterson, and Bogaert (2002) found that one in seven homosexual males had large numbers of older brothers, indicating that another factor must be at work. The late birth effect for homosexuality appears not to be culturally dependent. Poasa, Blanchard, and Zucker (2004) confirmed the effect for Samoan homosexual males.

6.2 PRENATAL DRUG EXPOSURE AND TSTG

There is suggestive evidence that prenatal drug administration can trigger epigenetic mechanisms that result in TSTG. Specifically **antiepileptic drugs** (AEDs) and **diethylstilbestrol** (DES) are suspected, although the evidence is not conclusive because of limited data. Both of these drugs were involved in pharmaceutical accidents before it was determined that they harmed developing fetuses when given to a pregnant mother. In the case of DES, the harm from mutations extends into at least the third generation.

There is evidence that prenatal antiepileptic drug exposure may be associated with TSTG. Dessens et al. (1999) sampled adults whose mothers had taken either phenobarbital or phenytoin (Dilantin) or both during pregnancy. Of 147 subjects (72 male and 75 female), 1 was an MTF transsexual, and 2 were FTM transsexual. They performed statistical tests on these results to compare them with known population frequencies and obtained statistically significant results using population frequencies for MTF of 0.0084% and FTM of 0.033%. Although their exact statistical testing procedure is unknown, their statistical results would probably not be significant if they had used the population frequency rules of thumb selected in Chapter 3. They also found that those scoring highest on transgender rating scales were also in the group whose mothers had received prenatal AEDs. Hoenig and Duggan (1974) reported a case of transsexualism in which both the transsexual and her relatives showed epileptic symptoms. The epilepsy seemed to be transmitted through paternal lines. It is possible that the AEDs used to treat epileptic mothers during pregnancy were responsible for transsexualism observed in these studies.

AEDs have established effects in mutating and changing DNA expression (Holmes et al., 2001; Meisler & Kearney, 2005; Rosenberg, 2007; Waxman & Azaroff, 1992) including the two anticonvulsants involved in the Dessens et al. (1999) study. AEDs have been shown to trigger neuronal cell death in the brain during the prenatal period when neurons are normally proliferating (Forcelli et al., 2010). Hill, Wlodarczyk, Palacios, and Finnell (2010) reviewed the teratogenicity of AEDs and concluded that it doubled or tripled the incidence of congenital physical deformities.

Prenatal exposure to AEDs has been suggested as a potential mechanism for TSTG. Because of sample size in the Dessens study, the evidence is not conclusive. AEDs certainly affect DNA expression and mutation but so do other drugs, in particular, DES, discussed next.

It has been suggested that prenatal administration of the drug **DES** is a potential causal mechanism involved in MTF TSTG (Kerlin, 2005). The molecular shape of DES resembles that of estrogens, but the chemical behaves much differently from estrogens and has several deleterious nonestrogen effects. DES was prescribed in the United States and other countries to prevent miscarriages and for estrogen replacement therapy from 1941 through 1971 (Giusti, Iwamoto, and Hatch, 1995; Ibaretta & Swan, 2001; Swan, 2000). Humans were also potentially exposed through the food chain to DES because it was added to cattle feed and implanted in poultry during the period 1954–1972 (Raun & Preston, 2002).

DES is a potent chemical that penetrates the blood-brain barrier (unlike estrogens); its structure resembles that of an estrogen-like hormone, but some of its effects are clearly dissimilar from estrogens. It was prescribed for pregnant women until it was discovered that it had adverse teratogen (e.g., penis malformation) and mutagenic effects (e.g., female cancer) on developing children. DES was also shown to have effects on grandchildren, showing that its mutagenic effects transcend generations (Kalfa, Paris, Soyer-Gobillard, Daures, & Sultan, 2001).

When the adverse effects of DES were observed, epidemiological studies were undertaken to identify its effects and to create registries so that those exposed could be later tracked for future problems. Epidemiological studies did not look for or detect any involvement of DES with TSTG (Kester, Green, Finch, & Williams, 1980), and the Centers for Disease Control (CDC) and the National Cancer Institute (NCI) in the United States do not list TSTG as an effect of DES.

At the urging of participants at a CDC/NCI conference, Kerlin and Beyer (2002) and Kerlin (2005) conducted surveys through a website for males who had been exposed to DES in utero. More than 150 of the 500 males who registered on the site described themselves as transgender. At least 150 described themselves as TS pre- or post-GPS transsexuals. They comprised 90 transsexuals, 48 transgender, and 17 gender dysphoric respondents. Members also reported depression, anxiety, and eating disorders. For females exposed to prenatal DES, Ehrhardt et al. (1989) found that there was no FTM TSTG effect of DES.

The results of the Kerlin studies (Kerlin, 2005; Kerlin & Beyer, 2002) could be criticized because the sample size of DES-exposed sons (500) was small compared with the number of males who had been exposed. The best estimate that the CDC can make is that the number of males exposed was in the range of 1 to 3 million. The wide range of potential exposure to male children makes statistical analysis more difficult. The sample may also have been biased because DES sons with health problems may have been more attracted to the website/network than those DES sons without medical problems. Still, it was a positive response to the conclusions of the National Institutes of Health, CDC, and NCI that increased research on DES-exposed males is needed. To date, however, no additional studies have been reported for TSTG.

There are reasons to believe that DES does not act in a normal physiological way compared with endogenous hormones produced by the body. It does not bind to the main estrogen receptor and is an established mutagen and teratogen (van Gelder et al., 2010). DES effects increase the susceptibility to certain birth defects into the third generation, which clearly indicates a third-generation genetic mutation. It is considered a toxic chemical and a "hormonally active agent," and some of its effects, such as mutagenicity, are clearly not within the normal actions of hormones. It also acts to influence DNA expression (Block, Kardana, Igarashi, & Taylor, 2000). Because of findings that estradiol causes masculinization of reflex systems in the hypothalamus, DES feminization effects have to be regarded as nonphysiological, meaning that the effects do not occur in normal functioning. Researchers should be wary of DES as an experimental surrogate for estrogens.

There are larger, better characterized databases than the ones used by Kerlin and Beyer (2002) and Kerlin (2005), which could be used to study TSTG in DES-exposed males. The NCI and other organizations have access to a combined database of more than 5,000 females and 2,600 males who were exposed to DES. Although investigators have asked people in these registries about their sexual behavior (Titus-Ernstoff et al., 2003), they did not ask whether the people in the registry were TSTG. Udry (2003) criticized this study for not considering "gendered behaviors." Evidently none of the investigators involved in the Titus-Ernstoff study were aware of the Kerlin study, and as of 2012, no one has asked people in the DES composite registry whether they are TSTG (L. Titus-Ernstoff, Geisel School of Medicine, Dartmouth College, personal communication, 2012).

DES reduces right-handedness in males but has no effect on handedness in females (Titus-Ernstoff et al., 2003) based on self-identification of the hand used for writing. Using a more sensitive measure of handedness, the Edinburgh handedness inventory, Schachter (1994) found increased non-right-handedness attributable to DES in females. These findings will come into particular consideration in the next chapter because handedness correlates with TSTG and has both genetic and epigenetic causal factors.

Interpretation of all of the AEDs and DES studies are handicapped because of lack of control and/or knowledge of the actual drug doses received prenatally and, in the case of DES males, how many were actually exposed.

6.3 HANDEDNESS

As discussed in the next chapter, non-right-handedness is associated with TSTG. It is believed that genetics and epigenetics are dual causal factors in handedness, which serves as a potential model for a two-factor theory of TSTG. Because of this, discussion of handedness is deferred to the next chapter to avoid duplication.

6.4 PRENATAL CHEMICAL ENVIRONMENT AND MATERNAL STRESS

Prenatal exposure to toxic chemicals and maternal stress may be involved in epigenetic mechanisms for TSTG, although there are no direct effects established. However, we can outline some of the potential epigenetic mechanisms, including those that modify the androgen receptor (AR) gene, which is a genetic marker for MTF transsexualism.

The presence of chemicals found in our environment that might cause genetic mutation or mutation stress is well documented. As detailed in the study Environmental Chemicals in Pregnant Women in the United States (Woodruff, Zota, & Schwartz, 2011), the load of potential mutagenic chemicals in pregnant women is high and includes pesticides, fire retardants, PCB, BPA, and chemicals banned by the Environmental Protection Agency in 1979 but still in the environment. There are reports that common chemical pollutants modify the AR gene that contains a marker for MTF transsexualism. Chemicals that modify the AR gene include the herbicide linuron, metabolites of the fungicide vinclozolin, the insecticide methoxychlor, and the DDT metabolite DDE (Tamura et al., 2003).

Stress has been shown to cause changes in brain development (Braun & Bogerts, 2001), DNA mutation (Radman, 1999), and changes to gene expression (Massa Swanson, & Sharp, 1996). Recently it also has been shown that stress causes changes in RNA control of sperm synthesis that is transgenerational and results in changes in behavior in animals (Gapp et al., 2014). Supporting a potential maternal stress mechanism for TSTG is the finding that adoption is more frequent in transgenderism (Zucker, Lightbody, Pecore, Bradley, & Blanchard, 1998). The percentage of transgender children who were adopted earlier than 2 years of age was higher than those adopted later and control subjects. Pregnant mothers who are considering having their child adopted may be under stress. We know that psychological stress can cause DNA mutations and changes DNA expression (Kaiser et al., 2003) and early stress modifies brain frontal lobe neural density and complexity (Murmu et al., 2006).

6.5 PRENATAL TESTOSTERONE THEORY AND TSTG

There is a theory that postulates that extremes of endogenous prenatal testosterone levels in the developing fetus are causal mechanisms for TSTG. Although not referenced by a formal name, this **prenatal testosterone theory of transsexualism (PTTT)** is frequently referenced in presentations from medical health professions, the scientific community, and even by transsexuals and transgendered people themselves as the causal mechanism in TSTG. For this reason, it is important to examine the evidence for and against this theory.

The story of the PTTT begins, oddly enough, in California at the beginning of the 20th century. At that time, California was the center of the eugenics movement in the United States. The movement sought to prevent the inheritance of mental illness and low intelligence levels through sterilization mainly of institutionalized patients. In its day, this movement became quite popular nationally, with the support of the public and even scientific researchers. The movement was even supported by the Rockefeller and Harriman foundations. Supporting research was conducted at prominent universities and at the Cold Spring Harbor Institute. Joseph Mengele received funding to study eugenics in the United States from the Rockefeller Foundation before his subsequent infamous experimentation at Auschwitz. The movement continued in California until World War II, but by then the German Nazis had adopted and extended the eugenics philosophy to rid their country of "undesirable" genes. Some of their ideas came from the United States eugenics programs with additional inspiration came from the German biologist Ernst Haekel. Nazi eugenics activities expanded beyond sterilization to use eugenics as an argument for the murder of homosexuals, transsexuals, transgender people, Jews, and other groups of people.

After the end of World War II and the partitioning of Germany, the idea of eugenics was taken up in earnest by East German socialists. Their overseers in the Soviet Union also supported this idea, because people in the Soviet Union (and now Russia) are vehemently opposed to homosexuality and transsexuality in accordance with their prevailing culture. In response to this environment, some East German endocrinology scientists decided to find "humane" eugenic treatments to avoid the birth of homosexuals (Mildenberger, 2012).

While East German scientists were puzzling how to contribute to the government-supported eugenics movement, the **organization-activation theory of sexual behavior** (Org-Act) was being conceptualized (Phoenix, Goy, Gerall, & Young, 1959). The Org-Act was based on rat and guinea pig experiments. In research studies to test the theory, testosterone or other sex hormones were administered prenatally or to castrated animal rat newborns whose level of maturity was believed to approximate the maturity of prenatal humans (Diamond, 1960; Feder & Whalen, 1965; Harris & Michael, 1964; Neumann & Elger, 1966). The animals were then tested as adults with or without hormonal administration in situations in which they could have sex with an estrous female or sex-experienced male. If testosterone had been administered prenatally or in early life, it would then facilitate male rodent sexual behavior in adulthood even for early castrated animals. The results seemed to confirm that the sexual behavior of the animals was determined during early organization and activated by hormones in adulthood. Research to support the Org-Act concept continued in later studies (Dorner, 1967, 1988; Dorner, Götz, Rohde, Plagemann, Lindner, & Hartmut, 2001; Dorner, Poppe, Stahl, Kolzsch, & Uebelhack, 1991).

The Org-Act theory is a scientifically valid theory with regard to animal sexual behavior. However, the East German scientists extrapolated from the Org-Act theory and experiments to develop the theory that human homosexuality was a result of a deficiency in fetal testosterone levels for male children. The theory held that it could be avoided if mothers received testosterone augmentation during pregnancy.

Transsexualism was added to the homosexuality theory in 1988, and the PTTT was born. These scientists believed that MTF transsexualism resulted from fetal testosterone levels that were too low, and FTM transsexualism resulted from fetal testosterone levels that were too high. One need not practice sterilization or genocide; all one had to do to rid the population of homosexuality and MTF transsexualism was to inject pregnant mothers with testosterone.

The fall of the Berlin Wall resulted in German reunification and greatly reduced Soviet influence on science in the former East Germany research establishments. It was at that point that East German scientists publicly began to support rights for homosexuals (but they have not done so thus far with respect to transsexuals or transgender people). To date, there is no record that these or other scientists performed human experiments in which a pregnant mother was injected with testosterone to avoid homosexual or transsexual children.

6.5.1 Evidence Against the PTTT

Science indicates that the PTTT is unsubstantiated as shown by evidence coming from seven lines of evidence.

First, the Org-Act animal experiments on which the PTTT was based dealt with sexual behavior, not gender behavior. Sex and gender behavior are not the same, as was explained in Chapter 3. Animals engage in sexual behavior instinctively, usually triggered by pheromones released during female estrous. In humans, gender behavior is learned based on culturally devised gender behavior categories. Testosterone does influence the brain, but it seems to influence functions related to sexual behavior and aggression according to the aromatase theory, described later in the chapter (McCarthy, 2008).

Second, animals are incapable of having gender; at least they do not have sophisticated gender behavior categories like humans do. The animals involved in the Org-Act experiments were rats and guinea pigs, which are incapable of sophisticated gender behavior systems. Such systems required cognitive mechanisms beyond their capabilities. Only humans possess such systems (Meyer-Bahlburg et al., 2004). It may be possible for our anthropoid ape cousins to have a primitive form of gender behavior category, just as they have primitive forms of tool making and cooperative hunting. However, no animals have gender systems with the sophistication that human gender systems possess. Therefore we must conclude that the PTTT cannot be proved through animal experimentation.

A third blow to the PTTT is the discovery that during prenatal development, genes begin to form sex-specific brain reflex structures well before the gonads are mature enough to secrete sex hormones (Davies & Wilkinson, 2006; Dewing, Shia, Horvath, & Vilain, 2004). The original Org-Act theory does not allow for parallel genetic mechanisms for development of these sex reflex structures and would have to be changed (Arnold, 2009).

Fourth, nature has provided us with a "natural experiment" that tests whether low testosterone causes TSTG. **Kallmann's syndrome** is a phenomenon that is caused by a defect in the gene that controls expression of gonadotropin-releasing hormone. It results in low testosterone levels in males during the prenatal and adult period. According to the PTTT, low developmental levels of testosterone should result in high levels of MTF transsexualism. However, as of 2004, only 2 cases of Kallmann's syndrome have ever been reported to co-occur with MTF transsexualism in more than 50 years of worldwide reports (Meyenburg & Sigusch, 2001). Chronically low testosterone levels do not seem to produce MTF TSTG.

Fifth, the PTTT predicts that high levels of prenatal testosterone will result in increased frequency of FTM transsexualism. It turns out that nature has also provided a "natural experiment" test of this prediction. There are people conceived with an autosomal genetic DNA defect in the CYP21A2 area (6p31 chromosome location) that results in the phenomena of **congenital adrenal hyperplasia** (CAH; Vilain, 1998). This defect results in the adrenal glands secreting large amounts of testosterone starting prenatally. The genetic defect disrupts a brain-adrenal feedback loop that responds to the level of blood cortisol. Because the brain mistakenly senses that cortisol levels are too low, it keeps sending signals for the adrenals to secrete more cortisol. But this also results in release of testosterone from the adrenals. Once discovered, CAH is treatable with steroid hormones (e.g., betamethasone) that reduce the secretion of testosterone, but CAH is sometimes not detected in females until the absence of menarche is noted in late teenage years.

Female CAH brains are bathed in high levels of testosterone from an early prenatal age. Exposure to testosterone continues until they are treated.

If the PTTT were correct, one would expect that a large percentage of these females should be FTM transsexuals or transgender individuals, but this is not the case. As of 1996, there were no reports of a CAH female completing transsexual transition including genital plastic surgery (Meyer-Bahlburg et al., 1996). Of the more than 500 female CAH patients who have been reported in the literature (Berenbaum, Duck, & Bryk, 2000; Dessens, Slijper, & Drop, 2005; Dittman, Kappes, Kappes, Borger, & Stender, 1990; Hines, Brook, & Conway, 2004; Meyer-Bahlburg et al., 1996), only four have requested trans-sexual GPS masculinization surgery (Meyer-Bahlburg, et al. 1996). Many females with CAH are homosexual or bisexual (Dessens, Slijper, & Drop, 2005; Frisen, 2005; Hines, 2004; Money, Schwartz, & Lewis, 1984), as were these four females. The authors specifically reject classification of these four patients as having gender identity disorder or being transsexual based on patient confusion about their sex, gender, and sexual orientation. There is no record of whether these four actually completed FTM transition and genital plastic surgery (Meyer-Bahlburg et al., 1996). With regard to FTM transgen-derism there are only five other female CAH patients reported who could be considered as transgendered (Dessens, Slijper, & Drop, 2005; Froukje, Slijper, Stenvert, & Drop, 1998).

Assessments of the gender identity of CAH females does not indicate a masculine gender identity. When CAH females were asked, most surveys report satisfaction in a feminine gender role (Berenbaum & Bailey, 2003; Dessens, Slijper, & Drop, 2005). One study indicated a masculine gender iden-tity (Meyer-Bahlburg et al., 1996), but a later study led by the same author found no indication of a masculine gender identity (Meyer-Bahlburg et al., 2004).

We now know that testosterone does not act directly on the brain to induce male reflex and behavior organization. It turns out that estradiol actually produces male organization only where testosterone can be converted into estradiol. The **aromatase theory** indicates that this only occurs where the aromatase enzyme is present (McCarthy, 2008). Aromatase is an enzyme that catalyzes the conversion of testosterone into estradiol. It appears that the organization of the brain by estradiol influences parts of the brain that control sexual reflexes, aggression, and play behavior. Some CAH females do seem to prefer nontraditional play behavior, vocations, and avocations such as construction and sports (Berenbaum, Duck, & Bryk, 2000; Dessens, Slijper, & Drop, 2005; Hines, 2006; Servin, Nordenstrom, Larrsson, & Bohlin, 2003; Udry, Morris, & Kovenock, 1995) but, in modern times, such behaviors are not regarded as exclusively masculine in Western cultures. Presumably, such behavior is mediated by brain structures that are organized by estradiol.

Females with CAH have high levels of prenatal testosterone, but they tend not to have masculine gender identities and do not become FTM transsexuals or transgendered individuals in large numbers as might be expected from the large and continuous doses they receive, beginning in gestation.

Sixth, 2D:4D finger ratios are often cited as an indicator of the levels of prenatal testosterone, and they correlate with MTF and FTM TSTG (see Section 5.5). However, as noted previously in Section 5.5, 2D:4D finger ratio seems to have a high correlation with heritability, indicating that epigenetics play a minor role. Experimental and survey studies indicate a strong genetic influence on 2D:4D ratio. Although 2D:4D ratio is often cited as an indicator of the levels of prenatal testosterone, in fact, direct measurement of fetal prenatal testosterone is beyond the state of the art.

Seventh, although androgen insensitivity syndrome (AIS) research is often cited to support the PTTT because it results in low effectiveness of testosterone on cells, AIS is also associated with mutation of the AR gene which is involved in the formation of feminine gender predisposition. As described in Section 5.3, a feminine gender predisposition would account for the low frequencies of 46,XY AIS patients showing masculine behavior or requesting body changes to appear more male. Mutation of the AR gene is associated both with MTF feminization and with AIS, but MTF TSTG is not associated with AIS.

6.6 SUMMARY

This chapter has dealt with epigenetic mechanisms that might be involved with TSTG; Chapter 7 deals with phenomena in which the interaction of genetic and/or epigenetic mechanisms is suspected. Evidence of imprinting among TSTG stems from a high maternal aunt/uncle ratio. Some studies found that TSTG was associated with birth order and sibling sex ratio, which might indicate primary epigenetic mechanisms. However, other studies indicate that these family statistics are associated with homosexuality, not TSTG. It is well established that some epigenetic effects are caused by prenatal exposure to drugs and toxic chemicals. There is initial evidence that antiepileptic drugs and diethylstilbestrol are associated with TSTG. Other epigenetic mechanisms are the result of exposure to toxic chemicals or maternal stress but, except for AED and DES, these have not yet been associated with TSTG. The PTTT is commonly invoked as an epigenetic mechanism for TSTG. However, evidence does not support this theory. This theory cites animal experimentation as evidence, and animals do not have sophisticated gender systems like humans. Furthermore, these animal experiments involved sexual behavior, not gender behavior. "Natural experiments" indicate that neither very high (FTM) nor very low (MTF) prenatal testosterone levels are involved with TSTG.

Although initial research evidence of an epigenetic causal factor for TSTG is limited, it suggests that future research will be fruitful. Epigenetics is a young area of scientific study, and there are an increasing number of candidate mechanisms to explore.

REFERENCES

Arnold, A. (2009). The organization-activation hypothesis as the foundation for a unified theory of sexual differentiation of all mammalian tissues. *Hormones and Behavior, 55,* 570–578.

Berenbaum, S., & Bailey, M. (2003). Effects on gender identity of prenatal androgens and genital appearance: Evidence from girls with congenital adrenal hyperplasia. *Journal of Clinical and Endocrine Metabolism, 88,* 1102–1106.

Berenbaum, S., Duck, S., & Bryk, K. (2000). Behavioral effects of prenatal versus postnatal androgen excess in children with 21-hydroxylase-deficient congenital adrenal hyperplasia. *Journal of Clinical and Endocrine Metabolism, 85,* 727–733.

Blanchard, R., & Sheridan, P. (1992). Sibship size, sibling sex ratio, birth order, and parental age in homosexual and non-homosexual gender dysphorics. *Journal of Nervous and Mental Disease, 180,* 40–47.

Blanchard, R., Zucker, K., Bradley, S. J., & Hume, C. S. (1995). Birth order and sibling sex ratio in homosexual adolescents and probable prehomosexual feminine boys. *Developmental Psychology, 31,* 22–30.

Blanchard, R., Zucker, K., Cohen-Kettenis, P., Gooren, L. & Bailey, J. (1996). Birth order and sibling sex ratio in two samples of Dutch gender-dysphoric homosexual males. *Archives of Sexual Behavior, 25,* 495–514.

Block, K., Kardana, A., Igarshi, P., Taylor, H. S. (2000). In utero diethylstilbestrol (DES) exposure alters Hox gene expression in the delveloping müllena system. *The FASEB Journal, 14*(9), 1101–1108.

Bogaert, A. (2003a). Interaction of fraternal birth order and body size in male sexual orientation. *Behavioral Neuroscience, 117,* 381–384.

Bogaert, A. (2003b). Number of older brothers and sexual orientation: New tests and the attraction/behavior distinction in two national probability samples. *Journal of Personality and Social Psychology, 84,* 644–652.

Bogaert, A. (2004). The prevalence of male homosexuality: The effect of fraternal birth order and variations in family size. *Journal of Theoretical Biology, 230,* 33–37.

Braun, K., & Bogerts, B. (2001). Experience guided neuronal plasticity. Significance for pathogenesis and therapy of psychiatric diseases. *Der Nervenarzt, 72,* 3–10.

Bruder, C., Piotrowski, A., Gijsbers, A. A., Andersson, R., Erickson, S., Diaz de Ståhl, T., . . . Dumanski, J. P. (2008). Phenotypically concordant and discordant monozygotic twins display different DNA copy-number-variation profiles. *American Journal of Human Genetics, 82,* 763–771.

Cantor, J., Blanchard, R., Paterson, A., & Bogaert, A. (2002). How many gay men owe their sexual orientation to fraternal birth order? *Archives of Sexual Behavior, 31,* 63–71.

Davies, W., & Wilkinson, L. (2006, December). It is not all hormones: Alternative explanations for sexual differentiation of the brain. *Brain Research*, *1126*, 36–45.

Dessens, A., Cohen-Kettenis, P. T., Mellenbergh, G. J., v.d. Poll, N., Koppe, J. G., & Boer, K. (1999). Prenatal exposure to anticonvulsants and psychosexual development. *Archives of Sexual Behavior*, *28*, 31–44.

Dessens, A., Slijper, F., & Drop, S. (2005). Gender dysphoria and gender change in chromosomal females with congenital adrenal hyperplasia. *Archives of Sexual Behavior*, *34*, 389–397.

Dewing, P., Shia, T., Horvath S., & Vilain, E. (2004). Sexually dimorphic gene expression in mouse brain precedes gonadal differentiation. *Molecular Brain Research*, *118*, 82–90.

Diamond, M. (1960, July). Comparative behavioral and structural effects of androgen injected into pregnant and non-pregnant guinea pigs. *The Anatomical Record*, *137*, 349.

Dittman, R., Kappes, M., Kappes, M., Borger, D., & Stender, H. (1990). Congenital adrenal hyperplasia I: Gender-related behavior and attitudes in female patients and sisters. *Psychoneuroendocrinology*, *15*, 401–420.

Dorner, G. (1967). Animal experimental studies on the problem of the hormonal pathogenesis of homosexuality. *Acta Biologica et Medica Germanica*, *19*, 569–584.

Dorner, G. (1988, February). Neuroendocrine response to estrogen and brain differentiation in heterosexuals, homosexuals and transsexuals. *Archives of Sexual Behavior*, *17*, 57–75.

Dorner, G., Götz, F., Rohde, W., Plagemann, P., Lindner, R., & Hartmut, P. (2001). Genetic and epigenetic effects on sexual brain organization mediated by sex hormones. *Neuroendocrinology Letters*, *22*, 403–409.

Dorner, G., Poppe, F., Stahl, F., Kolzsch, J., & Uebelhack, R. (1991). Gene and environmental-dependent neuroendocrine etiogenesis of homosexuality and transsexualism. *Experimental and Clinical Endocrinology*, *98*, 141–150.

Ehrhardt, A. A., Meyer-Bahlburg, H. F., Rosen, L. R., Feldman, J. F., Veridiano, N. P., Elkin, E. J., & McEwen, B. S. (1989). The development of gender-related behavior in females following prenatal exposure to diethylstilbestrol (DES). *Hormones and Behavior*, *23*, 526–541.

Feder, H., & Whalen, R. (1965, January 15). Feminine behavior in neonatally castrated and estrogen-treated male rats. *Science*, *147*, 306–307.

Forcelli, P., Janssen, M. J., Stamps, L. A., Sweeney, C., Vicini, S., & Gale, K. (2010). Therapeutic strategies to avoid long-term adverse outcomes of neonatal antiepileptic drug exposure. *Epilepsia*, *51*(Suppl. 30), 18–23.

Frisen, L., Nordenström, A., Falhammar, H., Filpsson, H., Holmdahl, G., Janson, PO., Thorén, M., Hagenfeldt, K., Möller, A., Nordenskjöld, A. (2009). Gender role behavior, sexuality, and psychosocial adaptation in women with congenital adrenal hyperplasia due to CYP21A2 deficiency. *J Clin Endocrinol Metlab, 94*(9), 3432–3439.

Froukje, M., Slijper, E., Stenvert, L., & Drop, S. (1998). Long-term psychological evaluation of intersex children. *Archives of Sexual Behavior, 27,* 125–144.

Gapp, K., Jawaid, A., Sarkies, P., Bohacek, J., Pelczar, P., Prados, J., . . . Mansuy, I. M. (2014). Implication of sperm RNAs in transgenerational inheritance of the effects of early trauma in mice. *Nature Neuroscience, 17,* 667–669.

Giusti, R., Iwamoto, K., & Hatch, E. (1995). Diethylstilbestrol revisited: A review of the long-term health effects. *Annals of Internal Medicine, 122,* 778–788.

Gómez-Gil, E., Esteva, I., Carrasco, R., Almaraz, M. C., Pasaro, E., Salamero, M., & Guillamon, A. (2010). Birth order and ratio of brothers to sisters in Spanish transsexuals. *Archives of Sexual Behavior, 40*(3), 505–510.

Gordon, L., Joo, J. E., Powell, J. E., Ollikainen, M., Novakovic, B., Li, X., Andronikos, R., . . . Saffrey, R. (2012). Neonatal DNA methylation profile in human twins is specified by a complex interplay between intrauterine environmental and genetic factors, subject to tissue-specific influence. *Genome Research, 22,* 1395–1406.

Green, R. (2000). Family co-occurrence of "gender dysphoria": Ten sibling or parent–child pairs. *Archives of Sexual Behavior, 29,* 499–507.

Green, R., & Keverne, E. (2000). The disparate maternal aunt–uncle ratio in male transsexuals: An explanation invoking genomic imprinting. *Journal of Theoretical Biology, 202,* 55–63.

Harris, G., & Michael, R. (1964). The activation of sexual behavior by hypothalamic implants of estrogen. *Journal of Physiology, 171,* 275–301.

Hill, D., Wlodarczyk, B., Palacios, A., & Finnell, R. (2010). Teratogenic effects of antiepileptic drugs. *Expert Reviews in Neurotherapy, 10,* 943–959.

Hines, M. (2006). Prenatal testosterone and gender-related behaviour. *European Journal of Endocrinology, 155*(Suppl. 1), S115–S121.

Hines, M., Brook, C., & Conway, G. (2004). Androgen and psychosexual development: Core gender identity, sexual orientation, and recalled childhood gender role behavior in women and men with congenital adrenal hyperplasia (CAH). *Journal of Sexual Research, 41,* 75–81.

Hoenig, J., & Duggan, E. (1974). Sexual and other abnormalities in the family of a transsexual. *Psychiatr. Clin. Basel. 7*(6), 334–346.

Holmes, L. B., Harvey, E. A., Coull, B. A., Huntington, K. B., Khoshbin, S., Hayes, A. M., & Ryan, L. M. (2001). The teratogenicity of anticonvulsant drugs. *New England Journal of Medicine, 344,* 1132–1138.

Ibaretta, D., & Swan, S. (2001). The DES story: Long term consequences of prenatal exposure. In P. Harimose (Ed.), *European Environmental Agency Environmental Issue Report,* No. 22 (Chapter 8). Copenhagen: European Environmental Agency.

Kaiser, F., Kruijver, F. P., Straub, R. H., Sachser, N., & Swaab, D. F. (2003). Early social stress in male guinea pigs changes social behavior, and autonomic and neuroendocrine functions. *Journal of Neuroendocrinology, 15,* 761–769.

Kalfa, N., Paris, F., Soyer-Gobillard, M., Daures, J., & Sultan, C. (2001). Prevalence of hypospadias in grandsons of women exposed to diethylstilbestrol during pregnancy: A multigenerational national cohort study. *Fertility and Sterility, 95,* 2574–2577.

Kerlin, S. (2005). *Prenatal exposure to diethylstilbestrol (DES) in males and gender-related disorders: Results from a 5-year study.* Paper prepared for the International Behavioral Development Symposium 2005. Retrieved October 17, 2013, from http://e.hormone.tulane.edu.

Kerlin, S., & Beyer, D. (2002). The DES Sons online discussion network. *Transgender Tapestry, 100,* 18.

Kester, P., Green, R., Finch, S., & Williams, K. (1980). Prenatal female hormone administration and psychosexual development in human males. *Psychoneuroendocrinology, 5,* 269–285.

Massa, S., Swanson, R., & Sharp, F. (1996). The stress gene response in brain. *Cerebrovascular Brain Metabolism Review, 8,* 95–158.

McCarthy, M. (2008). Estradiol and the developing brain. *Physiology Review, 88,* 91–134.

Meisler, M., & Kearney, J. (2005). Sodium channel mutations in epilepsy and other neurological disorders. *Journal of Clinical Investigation, 115,* 2010–2017.

Meyenburg, B., & Sigusch, V. (2001). Kallmann syndrome and transsexualism. *Archives of Sexual Behavior, 30,* 75–81.

Meyer-Bahlburg, H., Dolezal, C., Baker, S., Carlson, A., Obeid, J., & New, M. (2004). Prenatal androgenization affects gender-related behavior but not gender identity in 5-12-year-old girls with congenital adrenal hyperplasia. *Archives of Sexual Behavior, 33,* 97–104.

Meyer-Bahlburg, H., Feldman, J., Cohen, P., & Ehrhardt, A. (1988). Perinatal factors in the development of gender related play: Sex hormones versus pregnancy complications. *Psychiatry, 51,* 260–271.

Meyer-Bahlburg, H., Gruen, R. S., New, M. I., Bell, J. J., Morishima, M. S., Bueno, Y., Vargas, H., Baker, S. W. (1996). Gender change from female to male in classical congenital adrenal hyperplasia. *Hormones and Behavior, 30(4),* 319–332.

Mildenberger, F. (2012). Socialist eugenics and homosexuality in the GDR: The case of Günter Dörner. In S. Spector, H. Puff, & D. Herzog (Eds.), *After the history of sexuality: German genealogies with and beyond Foucault* (Vol. 5 of the Spectrum series). New York: Berghahn Books.

Money, J., Schwartz, M., & Lewis, V. (1984). Adult erotosexual status and fetal hormonal masculinization and demasculinization: 46,XX congenital virilizing adrenal hyperplasia and 46,XY androgen-insensitivity syndrome compared. *Psychoneuroendocrinology, 9,* 405–414.

Murmu, M., Salomon, S., Biala, Y., Weinstock, M., Braun, K., & Bock, J. (2006). Changes of spine density and dendritic complexity in the prefrontal cortex in offspring of mothers exposed to stress during pregnancy. *European Journal of Neuroscience, 24,* 1477–1487.

Neumann, F., & Elger, W. (1966). Permanent changes in gonadal function and sexual behavior as a result of early feminization of male rats by treatment with an antiandrogenic steroid. *Endokrinologie, 50,* 209–224.

Phoenix, C., Goy, R., Gerall, A., & Young, W. (1959). Organizing action of prenatally administered testosterone proportionate on the tissues mediating mating behavior in the female guinea pig. *Endocrinology, 65,* 369–382.

Poasa, K., Blanchard, R., & Zucker, K. (2004). Birth order in transgendered males from Polynesia: A quantitative study of Samoan Fa'afafine. *Journal of Sex & Marital Therapy, 30,* 13–23.

Radman, M. (1999). Mutations: Enzymes of evolutionary change. *Nature,* 401, 866–869.

Raun, A., & Preston, R. (2002). History of diethylstilbestrol use in cattle. *American Society for Animal Science.* Retrieved February 25, 2014, from https://www.asas.org/docs/publications/raunhist.pdf?sfvrsn=0.

Rosenberg, G. (2007). The mechanisms of action of valproate in neuropsychiatric disorders: Can we see the forest for the trees? *Cellular and Molecular Life Sciences, 64,* 2090–2103.

Schachter, S. (1994). Handedness in women with intrauterine exposure to diethylstilbestrol. *Neuropsychologia, 32,* 619–623.

Schagen, S., Delemarre-van de Waal, H. A., Blanchard, R., & Cohen-Kettenis, P. T. (2012). Sibling sex ratio and birth order in early-onset gender dysphoria. *Archives of Sexual Behavior, 41,* 541–549.

Servin, A., Nordenstrom, A., Larrsson, A., & Bohlin, G. (2003). Prenatal androgens and gender-typed behavior: A study of girls with mild and severe forms of congenital adrenal hyperplasia. *Developmental Psychology, 39,* 440–450.

Swan, S. (2000). Intrauterine exposure to diethylstilbestrol: Long-term effects in humans. *Acta Pathologica Microbiologica et Immunologica Scandinavica, 108,* 793–804.

Tamura, H., Yoshikawa, H., Gaido, K. W., Ross, S. M., DeLisle, R. K., Welsh, W. J., & Richard, A. M. (2003). Interaction of organophosphate pesticides and related compounds with the androgen receptor. *Environmental Health Perspectives, 111,* 545–552.

Titus-Ernstoff, L., Perez, K., Hatch, E. E., Troisi, R., Palmer, J. R., Hartge, P., . . . Hoover, R. (2003). Psychosexual characteristics of men and women exposed prenatally to diethylstilbestrol. *Epidemiology, 14,* 155.

Udry, J., Morris, N., & Kovenock, J. (1995). Androgen effects on women's gendered behavior. *Journal of Biosocial Science, 27,* 359–368.

Udry, R. (2003). Putting prenatal effects of sex-dimorphic behavior in perspective: An absolutely complete theory. *Epidemiology, 14,* 135.

van Gelder, M. M., van Rooij, I. A., Miller, R. K., Zielhuis, G. A., de Jong-van den Berg, L. T., & Roeleveld, N. (2010, July). Teratogenic mechanisms of medical drugs. *Human Reproduction Update, 16,* 378–394.

Vilain, E. (1998). CYPs, SNPs, and molecular diagnosis in the post-genomic era. *Clinical Chemistry, 44,* 2403–2404.

Waxman D. J., & Azaroff, L. (1992). Phenobarbital induction of cytochrome P-450 gene expression. *Biochemistry Journal, 281,* 577–592.

Woodruff, T., Zota, A., & Schwartz, J. (2011). Environmental chemicals in pregnant women in the United States: NHANE 2003–2004. *Environmental Health Perspectives, 119,* 878–885.

Zucker, K., Blanchard, R., Kim, T., Pae, C., & Lee, C. (2007). Birth order and sibling sex ratio in homosexual transsexual in South Korean men: Effects of the male-preference stopping rule. *Psychiatry and Clinical Neuroscience, 61,* 529–533.

Zucker, K., Bradley, S. J., Oliver, G., Blake, J., Fleming, S., & Hood, J. (1996). Psychosexual development of women with congenital adrenal hyperplasia. *Hormones and Behavior, 30,* 300–318.

Zucker, K., Green, R., Coates, S., Zuger, B., Cohen-Kettenis, P. T., Zecca, G. M., . . . Blanchard, R. (1997). Sibling sex ratio of boys with gender identity disorder. *Journal of Child Psychology and Psychiatry, 38,* 543–551.

Zucker, K., Lightbody, S., Pecore, K., Bradley, S., & Blanchard, R. (1998). Birth order in girls with gender identity disorder. *European Journal of Child and Adolescent Psychiatry, 7,* 30–35.

7

The Two-Factor Theory of Transsexualism and Transgenderism Causation

7.0 INTRODUCTION

The objective of this chapter is to synthesize information on the biological causes of transsexualism and transgenderism (TSTG) at the top level by proposing a two-factor theory of TSTG causation and presenting evidence that supports this theory. The theory relies on the definitions provided in Chapter 3. It also relies on the ubiquitous historical and geographic record of the existence of a biological gender predisposition as presented in Chapter 4 and the biological causal factors of genetics and epigenetics described in Chapters 5 and 6.

The **two-factor theory of TSTG causation** states that genetic and epigenetic causative factors are responsible for the phenomenon of TSTG. TSTG can result from genetics alone, from epigenetic mutations of DNA genetics, or from epigenetic influences on DNA expression. Although the genetics causal factor is statistically strong, there is still unaccounted for variance that could be attributed to epigenetics. As explained in Chapter 8, TSTG is not due to childrearing. At this time, TSTG cannot easily be traced through genealogy and family trees, which makes it more likely that epigenetics could be responsible for some instances of TSTG when there is no obvious inherited trait. Because molecular genetics and epigenetics are relatively young sciences, we do not have a complete picture of the alternative mechanisms that might be involved in TSTG, but this chapter discusses some of the possibilities to stimulate both thought and research.

7.1 SUPPORT FOR THE TWO-FACTOR THEORY OF TSTG CAUSATION

Support for the two-factor theory includes the following:

- Timing of the emergence of TSTG is compatible with activity of genetics and epigenetics factors
- Evidence of genetics and epigenetics involvement in TSTG presented in the preceding two chapters
- Heritability evidence and an existence proof of DNA markers for TSTG from Chapter 5
- The need for at least two factors to explain why genetics does not account for all of the variance heritability studies from Chapter 5
- Absence of proof for some causation theories and mechanisms (Chapters 8, 9, 11, 12)
- The lack of scientific formulation of psychodynamic theories that makes them empirically untestable (Chapter 12)
- Existence of potentially analogous two-factor theories that explain other biological phenomena that co-occur with TSTG, such as human handedness and certain biomarkers
- Existence of potentially analogous two-factor theories for certain human medical conditions with empirical evidence

An overview of each of these is provided in turn. Subsequent sections of this chapter provide more detail.

After mastering the fundamentals of gender behavior categories by age 2, (Poulin-Dubois, Serbin, Eighstedt, & Sen, 2002), TSTG typically starts to emerge by age 4. It appears that whatever causes TSTG, it must be present at birth or shortly thereafter, leaving little time for causal factors other than genetics and epigenetics to work. Genetics and epigenetics start working at conception and continue throughout gestation.

Child rearing does not seem to be a causative factor in TSTG, as described in Chapter 8. TSTG children appear able to readily learn gender behavior rules (Chiu et al., 2006; Maccoby, 1998; Szkrybalo & Ruble, 1999). It is true that parents do abuse transsexual and transgender children (Bandini et al., 2011; Koken, Bimbi, & Parsons, 2009), but the abuse is probably because of parents' intolerance of TSTG behavior. Improper parenting or parent interaction likely does not cause TSTG.

Chapters 5 and 6 on genetics and epigenetics provide evidence that each of these factors is involved in TSTG.

The heritability and genetic marker evidence from Chapter 5 implicate a genetics factor in TSTG. The heritability evidence indicates, however, that other factors may be involved in TSTG. The statistical inheritability loadings are strong but not as strong as body height and other traits.

The presence of genetic markers is an existence proof that some DNA genes are involved in TSTG. However, a full DNA scan is needed because many phenomena linked to genetics require multiple sites on the DNA molecule.

Subsequent chapters deal with other potential causative factors for TSTG. The evidence in these chapters eliminates these factors from current consideration. They include childrearing, sexual arousal, and homosexuality. Chapter 12 covers some historical psychodynamic theories that may be useful to clinicians but are not empirically testable. They therefore do not provide scientific evidence germane to TSTG causation.

Non–right-handedness is linked to TSTG in that both genetic and epigenetic causal factors are involved because they share a same genetic marker, and they are both influenced by prenatal exposure to certain of the same drugs. Transsexuals are known to be less right-handed than other people (Green & Young, 2001). As further explained in Section 7.2 later in the chapter, people fall onto a spectrum from right- to left-handedness, depending on the number of tasks they execute with a given hand. So it is not strictly correct to say that a person is right- or left-handed except when they use one hand for all tasks, which occurs rarely in the population. The current prevailing theory of handedness (Corballis, 1997, 2003; Corballis, Lee, McManus, & Crow, 1996) involves both genetic and mutation mechanisms. Corballis believes that a de novo mutation may be involved, but the evidence cited in Section 7.2 indicates that epigenetics mutations are involved.

In a large-scale study of more than 25,000 families, Medland et al. (2009) found that genetic influences account for 24.6% of the variance in handedness, with the remaining variance resulting from nonshared environmental influences. Finally, there are several phenomena that have been linked to a combination of genetic and epigenetic mechanisms. One of these, autism spectrum disorder, has been weakly linked to TSTG. The relationship between TSTG and autism spectrum are discussed in Sections 7.3 and 7.4. Potential two-factor theory mechanisms and their relationship are discussed in Section 7.5.

7.2 HANDEDNESS AND TSTG

The science pertaining to handedness is important to an understanding of TSTG because there are several studies showing that transsexuals are less right-handed than nontranssexual and nontransgendered people. Investigators have suggested that TSTG and handedness might have a similar origin (Ellis & Ebertz, 1997). Handedness refers to hand preference for various tasks, such as writing, drawing, brushing teeth, and so on. Few people are totally left or right handed. Most people fall on a continuum between left and right hands as to the number of preferred tasks per hand. Some investigators just ask which hand a person writes with, but others use a more sophisticated scale such as the Edinburgh Handedness Inventory, which measures 20 common tasks.

There are several reports of increased non-right-handedness among transsexuals in the scientific literature beginning with the first report by Watson and Coren (1992). Orlebeke, Boomsma, Gooren, Verschoor, and Van Den Bree (1992) found that a combined clinical sample of both male-to-female (MTF) and female-to-male (FTM) transsexuals from the Netherlands had a statistically significantly (8%) higher frequency of left-handedness using a 6-point behavior scale as a measure. The scale assessed writing, throwing, cutting with scissors, teeth brushing, drawing, and foot preference for kicking a ball. The samples of MTF and FTM separately were not statistically tested for male and female populations of left-handedness, respectively. Green and Young (2001) conducted a study in the United Kingdom using a similar scale to Orlebeke et al. (1992). Both MTF and FTM transsexuals were more often non-right-handed than control groups, respectively, of male and female subjects. Zucker, Beaulier, Bradley, Grimshaw, and Wilcox (2001) found increased left-handedness in a clinical population of transgender boys compared with control groups by 7% to 11%. Wisniewski, Prendeville, and Cobs (2009) observed a tendency for MTF to be less right-handed.

Non-right-handedness is linked to TSTG in that both genetic and epigenetic causal factors are involved, because they share a same genetic marker and are both influenced by exposure to certain of the same drugs. Medland et al. (2005) found a genetic marker for non-right-handedness on the androgen receptor (AR) testosterone receptor in the X chromosome. Note that this is the same location for the MTF AR TSTG marker as discussed in Chapter 5 (Hare et al., 2009; Henningsson et al., 2005). This marker is actually well researched and common to many phenomena including hypospadias, breast tumors (Gottlieb et al., 2013; Song et al., 2012), spontaneous preterm birth (Karajalainen et al., 2012), and now TSTG. These phenomena also include Kennedy's disease (Zajac & Fui, 2012), or spinobulbar atrophy, which is an X-linked inheritable disease. The CAG-repeat polymorphism is due to "slippage" during DNA replication. The slippage is caused by a temporary pause in DNA replication. High numbers of repeats are associated with TSTG.

Although TSTG and non-right-handedness share the same genetic marker, it must be kept in mind that most traits involve multiple DNA sites. Full DNA scans have not been performed for either TSTG or handedness. The motivation for looking at this DNA location for a handedness marker came from evidence that males have higher levels of testosterone and are more likely to be non-right-handed.

Because the heritability of handedness is only 24% to 26% (McManus, 2003; Medland et al., 2009) there must be epigenetic mechanisms at work. Epigenetic exposure to toxic drugs such as **antiepileptic drugs** (AEDs; Meador et al., 2013) and **diethylstilbestrol** (DES; Schachter, 1994) have been observed to increase non-right-handedness. Note that these two drugs are believed to be involved in prenatal epigenetic mechanisms involved in TSTG (see Section 6.2). Unrelated to TSTG and handedness, exposure to toxic chemicals such as DDE (a degreasing agent) has been correlated with increased AR CAG repeats (Bjork et al., 2011), indicating how genetic and epigenetic mechanisms may interact.

DES has been associated with TSTG (see Section 6.4) and DES has been shown to increase non–right-handedness in males but has no effect on females based on self-identification of the hand used for writing (Titus-Ernstoff, et al., 2003). Using a more sensitive measure of handedness, the Edinburgh Handedness Inventory, Schachter (1994) found increased non–right-handedness due to DES in females. DES exposure was implicated as a potential mechanism in TSTG in Section 6.3.

In summary, TSTG and handedness share a similar causal model involving the two factors of genetics and epigenetics, a similar genetic marker on the DNA locus expressed as the testosterone receptor, and association with DES exposure. These findings support the two-factor theory of TSTG.

7.3 AUTISM SPECTRUM

TSTG behavior has been reported in 6.0% to 7.8% of those who are in the autistic spectrum (AS). People in the AS have neurodevelopmental traits that cause social and communication deficits and stereotyped behaviors of varying severity. The overlap between TSTG and AS could be due to people with autistic traits being more open about their preferred gender behavior category. People in the AS are less sensitive to the reactions of other and they are thus less likely to fear discovery as TSTG. Whether or not the two phenomena are causally connected, the AS provides yet another example of how complex traits frequently involve both genetic and epigenetic causal factors. The population frequency of AS is approximately 2% (Blumberg et al., 2013) and involves the behavioral traits of difficulty in social interactions, difficulties in understanding other people's feelings, problems in speech and language comprehension, and behavioral obsessiveness.

There are several isolated clinical reports of the co-occurrence of TSTG and AS disorder beginning with incidental reports of small groups of patients. Williams, Allard, and Sears (1996) found two male children with AS disorder who were preoccupied by transgenderism. There was also a report of a single female who was both transsexual and in the AS (Landen & Rasmussen, 1997). A third incidental report was published regarding two male children with high-functioning AS disorder and also transgender (Mukaddes, 2002). Finally, Kraemer, Delsignore, Gundelfinger, Schnyder, and Hepp (2005) described a female who was transgender and also AS.

Group studies began with Abelson (1981) using the Michigan Gender Identity Test (Dull et al., 1975), which was validated on 30 children with autism and correlated with developmental scales. In a larger sample of 333 children, Noens et al. (2009) documented a clinical co-occurrence rate of 6% of people who were both transgender and in the AS. In a more systematic study, deViries, Noens, Cohen-Kettenis, Berckelaer-Onnes, and Doreleijers (2010) found a co-occurrence rate of 7.8% based on assignment of transgenderism and an AS test. Jones et al. (2012) found that FTM transsexuals had more autistic traits than control males, females, and transwomen. However, the FTM transsexuals had fewer autistic traits than an AS control group. In an adult population, Pasterski, Gilligan, and Curtis (2013) administered the Autism Spectrum Quotient scale and found that there were no differences among MTF transsexuals, FTM transsexuals, and control subjects. Of possible significance in the latter study was that all of the data used in the analysis were for nonhomosexuals.

Because the population frequency of transgenderism is at least 1% and probably higher and the population frequency of AS is 2%, it is possible that the observed co-occurrences of TSTG and AS disorder in clinical populations are by chance. The co-occurrence of two phenomena might also make parents more likely to bring children to an AS or TSTG clinic, thereby increasing the observed clinical co-occurrence rate. Another possible interpretation is that AS children and adults are more likely to reveal their TSTG because they are insensitive to others' reactions, which is an integral feature of AS disorder. They cannot feel the cultural rejection of TSTG. A third explanation is that TSTG becomes one of the forms of stereotype behavior.

In any event, AS provides a second model in addition to handedness for a two-factor theory of TSTG. AS has both genetic and epigenetic causal factors and mechanisms (Marchant & Robert, 2009). Heritability estimates from identical twins indicate a concordance rate of 60% for AS (Bailey, 1995). Chromosomal rearrangements have been observed, resulting in mosaicism (Jacquemont et al., 2006). Markers indicating increased likelihood of AS genes have been found on the fragile X DNA site (FMR1; Schaefer & Lutz, 2006) and several other sites (Marchant & Robert, 2009). Genetic mechanisms include de novo genetic mutation (Abrahams & Geschwind, 2008; Lintas & Persico, 2009; Michaelson et al., 2012; Sanders et al., 2012) genetic defects in mitochondria DNA (Napoli et al., 2012). Investigators are starting to conceive of

AS as involving a network of many protein-expressing genes that, if mutated, contribute to AS (O'Roak et al., 2012).

Numerous epigenetic mechanisms have been postulated for AS disorder, in part to explain the increases of AS disorder in the population observed over the past 3 decades. One of these could be classed as epigenetic imprinting in which the mother transfers non-DNA chemicals to her gestating fetus that interfere with brain development (Braunschweig et al., 2013).

7.4 OTHER ANALOGOUS PHENOMENA

Attention-deficit/hyperactivity disorder (ADHD) provides yet another example of how complex traits frequently involve both genetic and epigenetic causal factors. ADHD involves restless and impulsive behavior in both children and adults.

The ADHD model shares many of the features of the handedness and autism spectrum causal model: heritability, multiple genetic markers, and epigenetics (exposure to cigarette smoke in utero and other toxic substances) that interact with genes (Burt, 2009; Franke et al., 2012; Neale et al., 2010; Neuman et al., 2007).

Other phenomena involving both genetic and epigenetic causal factors include asthma and Down syndrome.

Note that mention of these phenomena is not to suggest a relationship with TSTG or that they are caused by the same mechanisms, but only that they are examples of phenomena that have both genetic and epigenetic causal factors.

7.5 POTENTIAL MECHANISMS OF TWO-FACTOR THEORY OF TSTG CAUSATION

The two-factor theory of TSTG causation summarizes the current scientific knowledge on TSTG and predicts that some combination of genetic and epigenetic mechanisms is responsible for TSTG. Identifying and characterizing these mechanisms and their interactions constitutes the next level of scientific understanding of TSTG. This is the next level of detail that should be pursued in the future. However, from current scientific evidence and analogous models of other phenomena such as handedness, we can identify some of the likely mechanisms.

From the existing scientific evidence, one can postulate that there is a network of genes responsible for gender predisposition. Most complex traits involve such networks of multiple genes, and even seemingly simple traits such as eye color involve 5 genes (Liu et al., 2009).

Then how is this gender predisposition genetic network tuned? Both genetic and epigenetic factors are involved. Some genes are passed on by parents without modification. A primary characteristic of the mechanism of direct inheritance is that traces of it should be found in family trees. However, there is little evidence that TSTG follows direct parental (Mendelian) inheritance rules. Both twin and nontwin siblings do share TSTG genetic inheritance. However, there are few reports of both male fathers and sons or female mothers and daughters both being TSTG. In the case of handedness, about 10% of the offspring of two left-handers become left-handed, and in the case of autism, parents typically have some of the same autistic traits as their offspring. For most other traits, parents would at least sometimes share the trait with their offspring if direct heritability were involved.

We might dismiss the lack of traceability from parents as the unwillingness of parents to reveal their TSTG, so we might expect more of these same-sex parent-child inheritances to appear as TSTG acceptance improves. On the other hand, genes for TSTG might come from the same-sex parent, which would be untraceable. Female mothers could pass feminine gender predisposition to their male sons, and male fathers could pass masculine gender predisposition to their female daughters. This would account for the absence of traceability because feminine gender predisposition in female mothers and masculine gender predisposition in male fathers would not be detectable. This means that TSTG genetic markers should be correlated with parents' DNA, especially same-sex parents.

We must also consider the possibility that TSTG is a form of diversity that creates the traits and skills within a clan or tribe that help ensure overall survival of the group. The two-spirit tradition lends support to this idea because many of the two-spirit individuals had skills from multiple gender behavior categories that were critical to a tribe. There is also a genetic mechanism called interlocus sexual conflict (Stulp, Kuijper, Buunk, Pollet, & Verhulst, 2012) that has been demonstrated in animals and newly demonstrated in humans. This mechanism occurs when a trait under selection from one parent constrains the other parent from passing on genes that might not be particularly optimal for survival of the individual but would be optimal for survival of the group. With respect to gender predisposition, this would mean that the maternal parent would pass on nurturing, feminine characteristics to her male offspring because this would lead to increased nurturing of offspring and thus increased survival of the tribe or group. Likewise, the paternal parent would pass aggressive masculine predisposition genes to daughters that result in improved warfare success and thus increased survival of the group.

Another potential mechanism that will also avoid parental and family traceability is a mutation of one or more of the parental genes before conception. This also could be observed by correlating TSTG genetic markers with parents. The prevailing theory of handedness specifies either direct inheritance or a mutation (Corballis, 1997). We need more research to determine when and how such mutations occur.

In Chapter 6, we identified several potential epigenetic mechanisms that could modify genes in the genetic predisposition network or change how they are expressed: imprinting, toxic drugs, toxic chemicals, and maternal stress. Imprinting involves passing on a chemical from a parent that can either protect or exacerbate the effects of a gene. Genetic repair mechanisms could account for the differences between identical twins if they both inherit the DNA for TSTG.

The interplay of genetic and epigenetic mechanisms could be detected by correlating not only the DNA genome but also what is now called the epigenome. The epigenome detects most genetic and genetic expression effects and is now within the state of the art.

7.6 SUMMARY

The purpose of this chapter was to organize scientific research findings on TSTG genetics and epigenetics causal factors by means of a two-factor theory of TSTG causation. There are other phenomena that involve both genetic and epigenetic mechanisms, notably handedness. Transsexual and transgender individuals are more non-right-handed than nontranssexual and nontransgender individuals. In addition, TSTG and handedness share a two-factor theory of causal factors, a common genetic marker, and a common correlation to AED and DES prenatal drug exposure. There are other phenomena that involve both causal factors such as AS disorder. Studies show that the co-occurrence of autism spectrum disorder and TSTG is 6.0% to 7.8%, but this could be due to the tendency of those with AS disorder to ignore or not understand other people's feelings about TSTG. The relationship between TSTG, AS disorder, and other phenomena does not imply that they share exactly the same mechanisms. There are several potential mechanisms that should be explored to provide more scientific detail for the two-factor theory of TSTG causation.

REFERENCES

Abelson, A. (1981). The development of gender identity in the autistic child. *Child Care: Health and Development, 7,* 347–356.

Abrahams, B., & Geschwind, D. (2008). Advances in autism genetics: On the threshold of a new neurobiology. *Nature Reviews Genetics, 9,* 341–355.

Bailey, A. (1995). Autism in a strongly genetic disorder: Evidence from a British Twin Study. *Psychological Medicine, 25,* 63–77.

Bandini, E., Fisher, A., Ricca, V., Ristori, J., Meriggiola, M., Jannini, E., . . . Maggi, M. (2011). Childhood maltreatment in subjects with male-to-female gender identity disorder. *International Journal of Impotence Research, 23,* 276–285.

Bjork, C., Nenonen, H., Giwercman, A., Bergman, Å., Rylander, L., & Giwercman, Y. L. (2011). Persistent organic pollutants have dose and CAG repeat length dependent effects on androgen receptor activity in vitro. *Reproduction and Toxicology, 32*, 293–297.

Blumberg, S., Bramlett, M. D., Kogan, M. D., Schieve, L. A., Jones, J. R., & Lu, M. C. (2013, March). Changes in prevalence of parent-reported autism spectrum disorder in school-age U.S. children: 2007 to 2011–2012. *National Health Statistics Reports, 65*, 1–11. Retrieved February 9, 2014, from http://www.cdc.gov/nchs/data/nhsr/nhsr065.pdf.

Braunschweig, D., Krakowiak, P., Duncanson, P., Boyce, R., Hansen, R. L., Ashwood, P., . . . Van de Water, J. (2013). Autism-specific maternal auto-antibodies recognize critical proteins in developing brain. *Translational Psychiatry, 9*, e277.

Burt, S. (2009). Rethinking environmental contributions to child and adolescent psychopathology: A meta analysis of shared environmental influences. *Psychological Bulletin, 135*, 608–637.

Chiu, S. W., Gervan, S., Fairbrother, C., Johnson, L., Owen-Anderson, A., & Bradley, S. (2006). Sex-dimorphic color preference in children with gender. *Sex Roles, 55*, 385–395.

Corballis, M. (1997, October). The genetics and evolution of handedness. *Psychological Reviews, 104*, 714–727.

Corballis, M. (2003). From mouth to hand: Gesture, speech, and the evolution of right-handedness. *Behavioral Brain Science, 26*, 199–208.

Corballis, M., Lee, K., McManus, I., & Crow, T. (1996). Location of the handedness gene on the X and Y chromosomes. *American Journal of Medical Genetics, 67*, 50–52.

deVries, A., Noens, I., Cohen-Kettenis, P., Berckelaer-Onnes, I., & Doreleijers, T. (2010). Autism spectrum disorders in gender dysphoric children and adolescents. *Journal of Autism and Development Disorders, 40*, 930–936.

Dull, C., Guiora, A. Z, Paluszny, M., Beit-Hallahmi, B., Catford, J. C., & Cooley, R. E. (1975). The Michigan gender identity test (MIGIT). *Comprehensive Psychiatry, 16*, 581–592.

Ellis, L., & Ebertz, L. (1997). *Sexual orientation: Toward biological understanding.* Westport, CT: Praeger.

Franke, B., Faraone, S. V., Asherson, P., Buitelaar, J., Bau, C. H., Ramos-Quiroga, J. A, . . . Reif, A.; International Multicentre Persistent ADHD Collaboration. (2012). The genetics of attention deficit/hyperactivity disorder in adults, a review. *Molecular Psychiatry, 17*, 960–987.

Gottlieb, B., Alvarado, C., Wang, C., Gharizadeh, B., Babrzadeh, F., Richards, B., . . . Trifiro, M. (2013). Making sense of intratumor genetic heterogeneity: Altered frequency of androgen receptor CAG repeat length variants in breast cancer tissues. *Human Mutations, 34*, 610–618.

Green, R., & Young, R. (2001). Hand preference, sexual preference and trans-sexualism. *Archives of Sexual Behavior, 30*, 565–574.

Hare, L., Bernard, P., Sánchez, F. J., Baird, P. N., Vilain, E., Kennedy, T., & Harley, V. R. (2009). Androgen receptor repeat length polymorphism associated with male-to-female transsexualism. *Biological Psychiatry, 65*, 93–96.

Henningsson, S., Westberg, L., Nilsson, S., Lundstrom, B., Ekseliusd, L. & Bodlunde, O. (2005). Sex steroid-related genes and male-to-female transsexualism. *Psychoneuroendocrinology, 30*, 657–664.

Jacquemont, M., Sanlaville, D., Redon, R., Raoul, O., Cormier-Daire, V., Lyonnet, S., . . . Phillipe, A. (2006). Array-based comparative genomic hybridization identifies high frequency of cryptic chromosomal rearrangements in patients with syndromic autism spectrum disorders. *Journal of Medical Genetics, 43*, 843–849.

Jones, R., Wheelwright, S., Farrell, K., Martin, E., Green, R., Di Ceglie, D., & Baron-Cohen, S. (2012). Brief report: Female-to-male transsexual people and autistic traits. *Journal of Autism and Developmental Disorders, 42*, 301–306.

Karjalainen, M., Huusko, J. M., Ulvila, J., Sotkasiira, J., Luukkonen, A., Teramo, K., . . . Hallman, M. (2012). A potential novel spontaneous preterm birth gene, AR, identified by linkage and association analysis of X chromosomal markers. *PLoS On, 7*, e51378.

Koken, J., Bimbi, D., & Parsons, J. (2009). Experiences of familial acceptance-rejection among transwomen of color. *Journal of Family Psychology, 23*, 853–860.

Kraemer, B., Delsignore, A., Gundelfinger, R., Schnyder, U., & Hepp, U. (2005, August). Comorbidity of Asperger syndrome and gender identity disorder. *European Child Adolescent Psychiatry, 14*, 292–296.

Landen, M., & Rasmussen, P. (1997, September). Gender identity disorder in a girl with autism—A case report. *European Child & Adolescent Psychiatry, 6*, 170–173.

Lintas, C., & Persico, A. (2009, January). Autistic phenotypes and genetic testing: State-of-the-art for the clinical geneticist. *Journal of Medical Genetics, 46*, 1–8.

Liu, F., van Duijn, K., Vingerling, J. R., Hofman, A., Uitterlinden, A. G., Janssens, A. C., & Kayser, M. (2009, March 10). Eye color and the prediction of complex phenotypes from genotypes. *Current Biology, 19*, R192–R193.

Maccoby, E. (1998). *The two sexes growing up apart, coming together*. Cambridge, MA: Harvard University Press.

Marchant, G., & Robert, J. (2009). Genetic testing for autism predisposition: Ethical, legal and social challenges. *Houston Journal of Health Law and Policy, 9*, 203–235.

McCarthy, M. (2008). Estradiol and the developing brain. *Physiological Review, 88*, 91–134.

McManus, C. (2003). *Right hand, left hand*. London: Phoenix.

Meador, K., Baker, G. A., Browning, N., Cohen, M. J., Bromley, R. L., Clayton-Smith, J., . . . Loring, D. W.; NEAD Study Group. (2013). Fetal antiepileptic drug exposure and cognitive outcomes at age 6 years (NEAD study): A prospective observational study. *Lancet Neurology, 23,* 244–252.

Medland, S., Duffy, D. L., Spurdle, A. B., Wright, M. J., Geffen, G. M., Montgomery, G. W., & Martin, N. G. (2005). Opposite effects of androgen receptor CAG repeat length on increased risk of left-handedness in males and females. *Behavioral Genetics, 35,* 735–744.

Medland, S., Duffy, D. L., Wright, M. J., Geffen, G. M., Hay, D. A., Levy, F., . . . Boomsma, D. I. (2009). Genetic influences on handedness: Data from 25,732 Australian and Dutch twin families. *Neuropsychologia, 47,* 330–337.

Michaelson, J., Shi, Y., Gujral, M., Zheng, H., Malhotra, D., Jin, X., . . . Sebat, J. (2012). Whole-genome sequencing in autism identifies hot spots for de novo germline mutation. *Cell, 151,* 1431–1442.

Mukaddes, N. (2002, November). Gender identity problems in autistic children. *Child Care Health and Development, 28,* 529–532.

Napoli, E., Ross-Inta, C., Hung, C., Fujisawa, F., Sakaguchi, D., Angelastro, J., . . . Ciulivi, C. (2012). Mitochondrial dysfunction in *Pten* haplo-insufficient mice with social deficits and repetitive behavior: Inteplay between *Pten* and p53. *PLoS ONE, 7,* e42504.

Neale, B., Medland, S. E., Ripke, S., Asherson, P., Franke, B., Lesch, K. P., . . . Nelson, S.; Psychiatric GWAS Consortium: ADHD Subgroup. (2010). Meta-analysis of genome-wide association studies of attention deficit/hyperactivity disorder. *Journal of the American Academy of Child and Adolescent Psychiatry, 49,* 884–897.

Neuman, R., Lobos, E., Reich, W., Henderson, C. A., Sun, L. W., & Todd, R. D. (2007). Prenatal smoking exposure and dopaminergic genotypes interact to cause severe ADHD subtype. *Biological Psychiatry, 15,* 1320–1328.

Noens, I., deVries, A., Cohen-Kettenis, P., Doreleijers, T., & Berckelaer-Onnes, I. (2009, May). *Co-occurrence of autism spectrum disorders in individuals with gender dysphoria.* Presented at the International Meeting for Autism Research, Chicago, IL.

Orlebeke, J., Boomsma, D. I., Gooren, L. J. G., Verschoor, A. M., & Van Den Bree, M. J. M. (1992). Elevated sinistrality in transsexuals. *Neuropsychology, 6,* 351–355.

O'Roak, B. J., Vives, L., Giriajan, S., Karakoc, E., Krumm, N., Coe, B. P., . . . Eichler, E. E. (2012). Sporadic autism exomes reveal a highly interconnected protein network of de novo mutations. *Nature, 485,* 246–250.

Pasterski, V., Gilligan, L., & Curtis, R. (2013, July). Traits of autism spectrum disorders in adults with gender dysphoria. *Archives of Sexual Behavior, 43,* 387–393.

Poulin-Dubois, D., Serbin, L., Eighstedt, J., & Sen, M. (2002). Men don't put on makeup: Toddlers' knowledge of the gender stereotyping of household activities. *Social Development, 11,* 166–181.

Sanders, S., Murtha, M. T., Gupta, A. R., Murdoch, J. D., Raubeson, M. J., Willsey, A. J., . . . State, M. W. (2012, April). De novo mutations revealed by whole-exome sequencing are strongly associated with autism. *Nature, 485,* 237–241.

Schachter, S. (1994). Handedness in women with intrauterine exposure to diethylstilbestrol. *Neuropsychologia, 32,* 619–623.

Schaefer, G., & Lutz, R. (2006). Diagnostic yield in the clinical genetic evaluation of autism spectrum disorders. *Advances in Autism, 549,* 367–372.

Song, Y., Geng, J.-S., Liu, T., Zhong, Z.-B., Liu, Y., Xia, B.-S., . . . Pang, D. (2012). Long CAG repeat sequence and protein expression of androgen receptor considered as prognostic indicators in male breast carcinoma. *PLoS One, 7,* e52271. Retrieved February 9, 2014, from http://www.plosone.org/article/info%3Adoi%2F10.1371%2Fjournal.pone.0052271.

Stulp, G., Kuijper, B., Buunk, A., Pollet, T., & Verhulst, S. (2012). Intralocus sexual conflict over human height. *Biology Letters, 8,* 976.

Szkrybalo, J., & Ruble, D. (1999). "God made me a girl": Sex-category constancy judgments and explanations revisited. *Developmental Psychology, 35,* 392–402.

Titus-Ernstoff, L., Perez, K., Hatch, E. E., Troisi, R., Palmer, J. R., Hartge, P., . . . Hoover, R. (2003). Psychosexual characteristics of men and women exposed prenatally to diethylstilbestrol. *Epidemiology, 14,* 155–160.

Watson, D., & Coren, S. (1992). Left-handedness in male-to-female transsexuals. *JAMA, 267,* 1342.

Williams, P., Allard, A., & Sears, L. (1996). Case study: Cross-gender preoccupations with two male children with autism. *Journal of Autism and Developmental Disorders, 26,* 635–642.

Wisniewski, A., Prendeville, M., & Cobs, A. (2009). Handedness, functional cerebral hemispheric lateralization, and cognition in male-to-female transsexuals receiving cross-sex hormone treatment. *Archives of Sexual Behavior, 34,* 167–172.

Zajac, J., & Fui, M. (2012). Kennedy's disease: Clinical significance of tandem repeats in the androgen receptor. *Advances in Experimental Biology, 769,* 53–68.

Zucker, K., Beaulier, N., Bradley, S., Grimshaw, G., & Wilcox A. (2001). Handedness in boys with gender identity disorder. *Journal of Child Psychology and Psychiatry, 42,* 767–776.

8

Childhood and Transsexualism–Transgenderism

8.0 INTRODUCTION

The purpose of this chapter is to provide scientific information pertaining to transsexualism and transgenderism (TSTG) childhood issues. Most transsexual and transgender people realize in childhood that they have been assigned to a gender behavior category that is incongruent with their gender predisposition. This realization occurs shortly after their acquisition of knowledge of the basic principles of gender.

Child rearing does not appear to be a causal factor in TSTG based on research studies that tested various hypotheses of how child rearing or parent-child interactions might have resulted in TSTG. There is no evidence that TSTG is caused by parental abuse, but there is evidence that parents do abuse some transsexual and transgender children because they react negatively to the violation of cultural norms.

The World Professional Association for Transgender Health (WPATH) provides guidelines for treatment of transsexual and transgender children. Parents now have three basic options to deal with their child's TSTG:

- Follow WPATH guidelines, including counseling and possible social transition during childhood.
- Follow WPATH guidelines and add hormonal treatment to block puberty.

- Provide "reparative-like" therapy that rejects the child's biological gender predisposition (which is ruled out by WPATH guidelines).

The "reparative-like" techniques used on transsexual and transgender children include **operant conditioning** and "jawboning therapy." Operant conditioning involves reward for behavior in incongruent gender behavior category and punishment for behavior in congruent gender behavior category.

The importance of early recognition and intervention for transsexual and transgender children is now realized. Providing early counseling is helpful to both parents and children in understanding TSTG. Some children are allowed to pursue a "**social transition**" in which they adopt the behavior of their congruent gender behavior category and informally change their names and presentations accordingly. Social transitioning is sometimes combined with medical treatments to delay puberty using blocking hormones. The practice of blocking puberty allows children to express themselves in the gender category that is more compatible with their gender predisposition until they are in a better position to decide whether to begin transsexual transition. Transition can be postponed until their late teens without incurring the unwanted effects of puberty including breast growth and voice change. Early intervention is undoubtedly due to improved understanding of TSTG among the medical and mental health communities.

8.1 GENDER LEARNING AND CONSTANCY

It is surprising how at an early age, children are very knowledgeable about gender and how young some children are when they realize that they are transsexual or transgender. Children grasp basic gender concepts by 18 months (Fausto-Sterling, 2012) and are knowledgeable of gender stereotypes in toys by age 2 to 3 (Serbin, Poulin-Dubois, Colburne, Sen, & Eichstedt, 2001). If their gender predisposition is congruent, they internalize their assigned gender behavior categories by age 3 (Fausto-Sterling, 2012). They quickly learn the basic expected presentations and behaviors for each gender behavior category that their culture offers. By 18 to 24 months, children generally recognize the stereotyped household tasks and tools associated with each gender category (Eichstadt, Servin, Poulin-Dubois, & Sen, 2002; Poulin-Dubois, Serbin, Eichstedt, Sen, & Beissel, 2002; Serbin, Poulin-Dubois, & Eichstedt, 2002).

Studies show that transsexual and transgender children appear to suffer no deficits in gender learning (Chiu et al., 2006; Maccoby, 1998). Many become keen observers of gender behavior so that they can pretend to follow their assigned gender behavior category to avoid rejection. Transsexual and transgender children are well motivated to learn the culturally assigned behaviors that are associated with their assigned gender behavior category.

They are well motivated by the threat of rejection by their families and culture. They secretively become "students of the game" and "role players" who learn even arbitrary gender behaviors even though they conflict with their gender predispositions. Through practice and correction, many transsexual and transgender people become very good at this pretending act to become perfect children in their parents' eyes.

Gender-stereotyped clothing can be easily recognized by children 5 to 10 years old (Albers, 1998). Even the severest critic of early gender learning believes that children are fully capable of making important decisions about gender at age 8 (Martin, 1993), which is just before puberty in females. Male puberty usually starts by age 10. Gender behavior learning continues during childhood.

The concept of gender constancy refers to the ability of a child to correctly identify the sex of individuals and themselves (Kohlberg, 1996). Of course, the child can only guess as to the sex of others based on their gender presentation and assuming cisgenderism. What used to be sex constancy has been morphed into "**gender constancy.**" The concept of gender constancy is difficult to define. Although several clinical tests have been developed, the concept "remains complex and somewhat elusive"(Szkrybalo & Ruble, 1999). The final stage of gender constancy is that of "**gender consistency,**" which usually occurs by 4 years old but sometimes does not occur even until after age 7 (Emmerich, Goldman, Kirsh, & Sharabany, 1977). Transsexual and transgender children have been found to score differently from control subjects on tests of gender constancy (Zucker, 1994). These were from a clinical sample of children aged 10 to 12. Zucker interpreted these results to indicate a developmental lag in gender learning, which contradicts other studies (Chiu et al., 2006; Maccoby, 1998). However, the test results are open to other interpretations because of the many inconsistent findings in the constancy literature (Szkrybalo & Ruble, 1999) and because clinical samples may be biased.

8.2 REALIZATION OF TSTG

Green (1976) found that the realization of TSTG typically starts when children are 3 to 4 years old. Subsequent retrospective studies have found that 50% of TSTG children come to that realization before age 6, with a peak at age 5 (Kennedy, 2008; Kennedy & Hellen, 2010). The average first age of cross-dressing was 8 years old, with 84% cross-dressing before leaving grammar school (age 11 to 12 in the United States).

Some children are aware that "something is wrong" at age 3 or 4 but cannot label the problem as TSTG related until much later, sometimes not until adulthood. Many may not know the words to describe their TSTG experience until about the age of 15, but this has decreased to about 9 years old during the past half century (Kennedy, 2008; Kennedy & Hellen, 2010). Some transsexuals and transgender people have a feeling that something is wrong but do not understand what it is until adulthood.

The first reaction of the transsexual or transgender child to realization of TSTG is that there is "something wrong" with them and that "God made a mistake." The overwhelming response to realization of TSTG is secrecy because children soon realize that they are different in a culturally unacceptable way. Only 31% tell their parents about their realization of TSTG (Kennedy, 2008; Kennedy & Hellen 2010). The children who express their realization of TSTG become instantly aware that they may be subject to rejection and bullying. Culture allows female-to-male (FTM) children to express themselves more freely as "tomboys," but even then only 33% of FTMs are allowed to present in androgynous or masculine style. Only 2% express their male-to-female (MTF) TSTG. Because of this secrecy, the great majority of transgender people are not ever treated clinically and, if they are, only to deal with cultural rejection or marital difficulties. This means that clinicians do not deal with most of the transgender subpopulations. Because of this situation, conclusions based on clinical data about TSTG are often in error such as was reported in Chapter 3 regarding the population frequencies of transsexuals and transgender people.

Secrecy in childhood can lead to secrecy in adulthood with adverse consequences (Kelly, 2002). TSTG sometimes only emerge after an existential crisis that may result from a family death or medical emergency (see Section 11.1).

Those children who reject secrecy and choose to express their TSTG behavior experience extreme family and cultural rejection. They may be encouraged by their parents to conform through gentle persuasion up through severe shaming and punishment and outright expulsion from the family. Most children, whose gender predisposition and expected gender behavior do not match, will learn how to pretend to follow the correct gender behavior norms for their assigned sex and keep their true feelings a secret.

8.3 PARENTAL INTERACTIONS AND TSTG CAUSATION

Several aspects of child rearing and parental interaction have been suggested to be related to the causation of TSTG. Scientific studies either refute or are inconclusive about these suggestions (Bailey & Zucker, 1995; Cohen-Kettenis & Gooren, 1999) as described in this section.

8.3.1 Emotional Relationships with Parents

It has been hypothesized that the primary cause of MTF TSTG is the disruption of normal emotional relations between parent and child (Ball, 1967;

Stoller, 1968). Abnormal emotional relations have also been suggested as a contributory cause of TSTG (Uddenberg, Walinder, & Hojerback, 1979). These investigators blamed TSTG on a distant father or one who is not available for gender teaching or emotional support. Stoller (1968) believed that the mothers of transgender children were more likely to marry distant husbands.

Buhrich and McConaghy (1978) found that there was no evidence of pathological relationships between transsexuals and their mothers that could account for MTF or FTM TSTG. They did find that there was a tendency for fathers to lack interest in their transsexual children, but this tendency held true in their studies for the fathers of homosexuals as well as transsexuals. Parker and Barr (1982) found that FTM transsexuals, when surveyed, scored their mothers the same as controls but they reported their fathers as more protective but less caring. Cohen-Kettenis and Arrindell (1990) obtained similar results for both FTM and MTF transsexuals in ratings data.

The results in this area of inquiry do not indicate that emotional disruption of families is associated with the causation of TSTG. The results observed could well reflect parents' reaction to transsexual and transgender children. Individual parents of transsexual and transgender children may be more distant out of ignorance, culture, and fear of seeing TSTG behavior by their children.

8.3.2 Prenatal Sex Preference of Mother

Buhrich and McConaghy (1978) suggested that a causal factor in TSTG might result from the mother of a transsexual or transgender child, originally wanting a different-sex child, the notion being that the mother would then treat that child differently. This notion was refuted by a study showing that there was no relationship between TSTG and a mother's preferred sex before delivery that was mismatched to the actual sex of the child (Zucker et al., 1994). Mothers do not make children transsexual or transgender, even if they wanted a child of a different sex.

8.3.3 Parental Separation

It was also suggested by Buhrich and McConaghy (1978) that paternal separation from children was a contributory cause of TSTG. Subsequent investigators have found no such relationship for absent fathers (Cohen-Kettenis & Arrindell, 1990; Freund, Langevin, Zajac, Steiner, & Zajac, 1974; Stevens, Golombok, Beveridge, & The ALSPAC Study Team, 2002). This was confirmed in nontranssexual/nontransgender children who were able to learn gender roles despite the absence of that father (Stevenson & Black, 1988).

8.3.4 Raising Child in Wrong Gender Category

The idea that a child can be raised in an incongruent gender behavior category and that such persons will remain in that gender behavior category is a staple of transsexual and transgender fantasy stories. "Petticoating" by mothers, aunts, and teachers as punishment is actually practiced on male children, although it seems not as frequently as in older times. Petticoating involves humiliation of males by forcing them to dress in feminine clothing in public or semipublic areas. Folklore has it that if petticoating continues, the male child will permanently adopt an adult feminine gender behavior category. The story varies with regard to the amount of cooperation by the male. There is no evidence that petticoating works as a mechanism for TSTG.

There are examples in which parents have attempted to raise male children in a feminine gender behavior category because of accident or a difference in sexual development after genital plastic surgery. However, the incidence of rejection is considerable. These resulted from surgical mistakes or surgery to form female genitalia due to **cloacal exstrophy** (a genetic malformation that results in the splitting of genitalia).

Two cases occurred in which surgical mistakes were made during circumcision resulting in loss of the penis for two male children. Follow-up surgery was performed to make their outer genitalia look like females. Health care professionals mistakenly told their parents that they would become women if raised that way. Both of these "experiments" resulted in rejection of gender rearing and, in one case, suicide (Bradley, Oliver, Chernick, & Zucker, 1998; Reiner & Gearhart, 2004). One of these cases was documented in the bestselling book *As Nature Made Him* (Colopinto, 2006).

Reiner and Gearhart (2004) conducted a study in which 14 male patients with cloacal exstrophy underwent surgery within 12 weeks of birth to simulate female genitalia. The study period ranged from age 5 to age 16. They were raised as girls by their parents. Of the 14 surgically assigned female patients, 8 spontaneously changed to a masculine gender category during the childhood, but 2 children surgically assigned as male did not change (Reiner & Gearhart, 2004). Nothing has been published on the behavior of these children in adulthood.

Children seem to be born with a gender predisposition that causes them to reject incongruent assigned gender behavior categories, although they seem to be able to live uncomfortably in an incongruent category for some time and revert later.

8.3.5 Parental Abuse and Violence

Because parents may reject the TSTG behavior of their children, they punish such children through verbal abuse, physical abuse, humiliation, and guilt

(Bandini et al., 2011; Gehring & Knudson, 2005; Roberts, Rosario, Corliss, Koenen, & Austin, 2012). Because of the rejection and abuse of transsexual and transgender children, many are forced from their homes and become homeless. The evidence for such parental behavior includes reports of abuse to transgender children of color (Koken, Bimbi, & Parsons, 2009). Roberts, Rosario, Corliss, Koenen, and Austin (2012) suggested that some transsexuals and transgender people suffer from post-traumatic stress disorder because of this abuse.

There is no scientific evidence to support the theory that TSTG is due to childhood trauma inflicted by parents, although this notion crops up in psychodynamic thinking and in the rationale for "reparative-like" therapy (see Section 8.6). It is true that parents and others do abuse transsexual and transgender children, but the abuse is a result of their intolerance of TSTG behavior. There is no evidence to support the notion that TSTG is due to parental abuse, but there is evidence that parents abuse their children because of their TSTG behavior.

8.4 TREATMENT OF TRANSSEXUAL AND TRANSGENDER CHILDREN

This section describes three strategies that the parents of transsexual and transgender children can follow for treatment of their children:

1. Follow WPATH guidelines, which include counseling and possible social transition during childhood.
2. Follow WPATH guidelines as in Strategy 1, and add hormonal treatment to block puberty. This is relatively new.
3. Provide "reparative-like" therapy that rejects the child's biological gender predisposition (this is ruled out by WPATH guidelines).

8.4.1 Treatment According to WPATH Guidelines

The guiding documents for treatment of transsexual and transgender children are the Standards of Care published by the WPATH (2013), and "GID in Children and Adolescents: Guidance for Management" by the Royal College of Psychiatry (2003). WPATH is the relatively new name of the Harry Benjamin International Gender Dysphoria Association, which has published treatment guidelines since 1980. A task force of the American Psychiatric Association has recommended that their association develop treatment guidelines, but so far none have been promulgated. The American Psychological Association is also in the process of developing treatment guidelines.

To summarize the WPATH treatment recommendations:

1. A diagnostic analysis of the transgender child should be conducted that also considers family function and issues the child is encountering at school and elsewhere. The diagnosis should also consider co-occurring mental health or medical problems of the child.
2. Encourage families, peers, and mentors to have an accepting and nurturing response to problems encountered by the transgender child.
3. Psychotherapy should be available to help the transgender child with the difficulties they may encounter.
4. Do not attempt to change the child's gender behavior and expression of identity to conform to the gender behavior category they were assigned at birth. Such treatment is ineffective and no longer considered ethical.
5. Provide support for the decision and the process of social transition to full expression of the desired gender behavior category of the child.
6. Irreversible body changes (e.g., genital plastic surgery) should not be undertaken until adolescence.

8.4.2 Social Transitioning with Puberty Delay

The second strategy for dealing with TSTG children is to follow the WPATH guidelines and add delay of puberty using blocking hormones. This strategy is relatively new. Physicians have begun delaying puberty for transsexual and transgender children before age 8 or 9 for FTM and age 10 to 11 for MTF before puberty begins (Kreukels & Cohen-Kettenis, 2011), although the practice is more frequent in teenagers who have already shown signs of puberty (Kreukels & Cohen-Kettenis, 2011). It is recommended that female children begin blocking hormones by Tanner Stage 2 of breast development, which can occur as early as 9 years old (WPATH, 2013). Most treatment plans involve both puberty blocking and social transition treatment, but some do not. The benefits of delaying puberty are that children have more time to explore their gender predisposition in a new gender behavior category and that delaying puberty supports childhood social transition.

The blocking protocol involves administration of **gonadotropin releasing hormone** (GnRH) agonists that down regulate and desensitize the GnRH receptors in the pituitary, preventing release of **luteinizing hormones** (LH) and **follicle-stimulating hormones** (FSH) that are involved in puberty. The GnRH receptors decrease in number, preventing normal initiation of puberty. GnRH is normally secreted by the hypothalamus and passed along to the pituitary but administration of the GnRH agonists prevents the hypothalamus from triggering puberty through release of LH and FSH.

Typical GnRH agonist drugs used are leuprolide, histrelin, and, in the Netherlands, triptorelin. A nasal spray of nafarelin can also be used. All of these are GnRH agonists used off-label vis-à-vis the U.S. Food and Drug Administration or other regulatory agency. The goal is to delay potentially unwanted development until the child and parents are able to make an informed decision as to whether to start transsexual transition with hormone therapy at approximately age 16 to 18 years.

Reports indicate that treatment with blocking hormones is safe and leads to better outcomes (Baudewijntje, Kreukels, & Cohen-Kettenis, 2011; Delemarre-van de Waal, 2013; Nakatsuka, 2013; Olson, 2012; Shumer & Spack, 2013). Delaying puberty in this way reduces anxiety in the transsexual or transgender child and allows for those children who change their minds about TS before starting transition (Steensma, Biemond, de Boer, & Cohen-Kettenis, 2011).

8.5 REPARATIVE-LIKE THERAPY TECHNIQUES APPLIED TO TRANSGENDER CHILDREN

Some unethical therapists do not follow the WPATH guidelines and treat transgender children with techniques similar to some of those used in reparative therapy for homosexuals. The scare tactic used by these therapists on parents is that the transgender child will grow up to become homosexual or transsexual as adults if not treated in this way. There is no evidence that such therapies permanently change behavior or that they prevent homosexuality or transsexualism. There is, however, evidence that reparative therapy for homosexuality has caused psychological and physical injury.

The techniques include operant conditioning that "shapes" behavior and "jawboning" therapy that verbally punishes expression of congruent gender identity and verbally rewards expression of incongruent gender identity. **Operant conditioning** is used to "shape" gender behavior using a system of rewards and punishments to encourage behavior associated with the assigned gender behavior category of the child. Simultaneously operant conditioning punishes behavior associated with the transgender child's congruent gender behavior category. For example, a child might receive a token when manifesting "appropriate" gender behavior, such as playing with an "appropriate" toy, and a token would be taken away for "inappropriate" behavior. For example, for MTF, the appropriate toy might be a toy truck and an inappropriate toy might be a doll. Tokens can later be exchanged for rewards and treats. These operant conditioning techniques are known as positive reinforcement and negative reinforcement. Parents are asked to enforce the operant conditioning system and to take away all toys, clothing, and other appurtenances that are not associated with the culturally assigned gender behavior category. Operant conditioning may help in initial learning of desired behavior but when the environment of the patient changes the behavior may not be maintained.

Because parents and therapists lose control of the environment as children move into puberty and adulthood, learned behavior in an incongruent gender behavior category may only be used to provide cover stories to protect TSTG behavior.

Talk therapy and jawboning are used to lecture the transsexual or transgender child and his or her parents on appropriate behavior for the child's assigned gender behavior category. There is no scientific evidence that withdrawal of a toy or other object, operant conditioning, or jawboning works to deter homosexuality or transsexuality in adulthood. Such reparative-like therapy treatment may cause psychological damage to the transgender child, just as reparative therapy does for homosexuals.

Apparent behavioral changes due to these "therapies" in transsexual and transgender children may be illusory. Therapists and parents may be fooling themselves. From an early age and into adulthood, transsexual and transgender children have been shown to be capable of learning and displaying the tasks involved in an incongruent gender behavior category to avoid rejection. In private or anonymously, they may continue to behave in their congruent gender behavior category. However, pretending to belong to an incongruent gender behavior category may become exhausting and cause psychological and physical damage (Kelly, 2002).

Several professional organizations, such as the American Psychiatric Association and the American Psychological Association, have, for several years, promised to provide treatment guidelines for transsexual and transgender children as WPATH has done (Byne et al., 2012). The American Psychiatric Association takes a neutral position, both allowing reparative-like therapy and encouraging the expression of transgender behavior. The WPATH guidelines reject reparative-like therapy (Byne et al., 2012), whereas the American Psychological Association rejects reparative therapy for homosexuality but has taken no position on transgenderism. However, on the basis of the inaction by the American Psychiatric Association and the American Psychological Association, some mental health professionals feel free to continue to practice such therapies on transsexual and transgender children despite WPATH rejection. There is no known therapy or other treatment that will make TSTG go away.

8.6 SUMMARY

The purpose of this chapter was to describe TSTG issues in childhood. It is in childhood that TSTG begins when children understand the basics of gender behavior categories and a little later realize that their gender predisposition is incongruent with their assigned gender behavior category. Child rearing does not appear to be a causal factor in TSTG based on studies that tested and invalidated various hypotheses involving the child rearing or parent-child interactions. There is no evidence that TSTG is caused by parents, but there is evidence that child abuse does take place when parents see and do not understand behavior incongruent with the child's assigned gender behavior category.

Parents currently have three options to deal with a transsexual or transgender child. They can (1) follow WPATH guidelines, (2) follow WPATH guidelines and add delay of puberty, or (3) subject the child to reparative-like therapies that might include operant conditioning and jawboning to discourage transsexual and transgender behavior including expression of "inappropriate" gender identity (which is rejected by WPATH but not by the American Psychiatric Association and the American Psychological Association). Such therapies are similar to reparative therapies for homosexuals that have been shown to be ineffective and injurious to patients.

REFERENCES

Albers, S. (1998). The effect of gender-typed clothing on children's social judgments. *Child Study Journal, 28*, 137–159.

Bailey, M., & Zucker, K. (1995). Childhood sex-typed behavior and sexual orientation: A conceptual analysis and quantitative review. *Developmental Psychology, 31*, 43–55.

Ball, J. (1967). Transsexualism and transvestism. *Australian and New Zealand Journal of Psychiatry, 1*, 188–200.

Bandini, E., Fisher, A. D., Ricca, V., Ristori, J., Meriggiola, M. C., Jannini, E. A., . . . Maggi, M. (2011). Childhood maltreatment in subjects with male-to-female gender identity disorder. *International Journal of Impotence Research, 23*, 276–285.

Baudewijntje, P., Kreukels, C., & Cohen-Kettenis, P. (2011, August). Puberty suppression in gender identity disorder: The Amsterdam experience. *Endocrinology Nature Reviews, 7*, 466–472.

Bradley, S., Oliver, G., Chernick, A., & Zucker, K. J. (1998). Experiment of nurture: Ablatio penis at 2 months, sex reassignment at 7 months, and a psychosexual follow-up in young adulthood. *Pediatrics, 102*, 1–5.

Buhrich, N., & McConaghy, N. (1978, June). Parental relationships during childhood in homosexuality, transvestism and transsexualism. *Australia and New Zealand Journal of Psychiatry, 12*, 103–108.

Byne, W., Bradley, S. J., Coleman, E., Eyler, A. E., Green, R., Menvielle, E. J., . . . Tompkins, D.A.; American Psychiatric Association Task Force on Treatment of Gender Identity Disorder. (2012, June). Report of the American Psychiatric Association Task Force on treatment of gender identity disorder. *Archives of Sexual Behavior, 27*, 1–30.

Chiu, S. W., Gervan, S., Fairbrother, C., Johnson, L., Owen-Anderson, A., & Bradley, S. (2006). Sex-dimorphic color preference in children with gender identity disorder. *Sex Roles, 55*, 385–395.

Cohen-Kettenis, P., & Arrindell, W. (1990). Perceive parental rearing style, parental divorce and transsexualism: A controlled study. *Psychological Medicine, 20*, 613–620.

Cohen-Kettenis, P., Delemarre-van de Waal, H., & Gooren, L. (2008). The treatment of adolescent transsexuals: Changing insights. *Journal of Sexual Medicine, 5*, 1892–1897.

Cohen-Kettenis, P. T., & Gooren, L. J. G. (1999). Transsexualism: A review of etiology, diagnosis and treatment. *Journal of Psychosomatic Research, 40*, 315–333.

Colopinto, J. (2006). *As nature made him: The boy who was raised as a girl.* New York: Harper Perennial.

Delemarre-van de Waal, H. (2013, June). *Hormone therapy to halt puberty safe, effective in transgender adolescents* [abstract #FP37-3]. Presented at the Endocrine Society Annual Meeting and Expo, San Francisco.

Devor, H. (1994). Transsexualism, dissociation, and child abuse: An initial discussion based on non-clinical data. *Journal of Psychology & Human Sexuality, 6*, 49–72.

Eichstedt, J., Servin, L., Poulin-Dubois, D., & Sen, M. (2002). Of bears and men: Infants' knowledge of conventional and metaphorical gender stereotypes. *Infant Behavior & Development, 25*, 296–310.

Emmerich, W., Goldman, K., Kirsh, B., & Sharabany, R. (1977). Evidence for a transitional phase in the development of gender constancy. *Child Development, 48*, 930–936.

Fausto-Sterling, A. (2012). The dynamic development of gender variability. *Journal of Homosexuality, 59*, 393–421.

Freund, K., Langevin, R., Zajac, Y., Steiner, B., & Zajac, A. (1974). Parent–child relations in transsexual and non-transsexual homosexual males. *British Journal of Psychiatry, 124*, 22–23.

Gehring, D., & Knudson, G. (2005). Prevalence of childhood trauma in a clinical population of transsexual people. *International Journal of Transgenderism, 8*, 23–30.

Green, R. (1976). One hundred ten feminine and masculine boys: Behavioral contrasts and demographic similarities. *Archives of Sexual Behavior, 5*, 425–446.

Kelly, A. (2002). *The psychology of secrets.* New York: Plenum.

Kennedy, N. (2008). Transgendered children in schools: A critical review of homophobic bullying: Safe to learn—embedding anti-bullying work in schools. *Forum, 50*, 383–396.

Kennedy, N., & Hellen, M. (2010). Transgender children: More than a theoretical challenge. *Graduate Journal of Social Sciences, 7*, 25–42.

Kohlberg, L. (1996). A cognitive analysis of children's sex-role concepts and attitudes. In E. Maccody (Ed.), *The development of sex differences*. Stanford, CA: Stanford University Press.

Koken, J., Bimbi, D., & Parsons, J. (2009). Experiences of familial acceptance-rejection among transwomen of color. *Journal of Family Psychology, 23*, 853–860.

Kreukels, B., & Cohen-Kettenis, P. (2011, August). Puberty suppression in gender identity disorder: The Amsterdam experience. *Nature Reviews Endocrinology, 7*, 466–472.

Maccoby, E. (1998). *The two sexes growing up apart, coming together*. Cambridge, MA: Harvard University Press.

Martin, C. (1993). New directions for investigating children's gender knowledge. *Developmental Review, 13*, 184–204.

Nakatsuka, M. (2013). Puberty-delaying hormone therapy in adolescents with gender identity disorder. *Seishin Shinkeigaku Zasshi, 115*, 316–322.

Olson, J. (2012, June 27). *Suppression of puberty in peripubertal transgender youth*. Center for Strengthening Youth Prevention Paradigms. Retrieved February 11, 2014, from http://lachildrenshospital.net/webinar/ DrOlsonConsultation/lib/playback.html.

Parker, G., & Barr, R. (1982). Parental representations of transsexuals. *Archives of Sexual Behavior, 11*, 221–230.

Poulin-Dubois, D., Serbin, L., Eichstedt, J., Sen, M., & Beissel, C. (2002, May). Men don't put on make-up: Toddlers' knowledge of gender stereotyping of household activities. *Social Development, 11*, 166–181.

Reiner, W., & Gearhart, J. (2004). Discordant sexual identity in some genetic males with cloacal exstrophy assigned to female sex at birth. *New England Journal of Medicine, 350*, 333–343.

Roberts, A., Rosario, M., Corliss, H., Koenen, K., & Austin, B. (2012). Childhood gender non-conformity: A risk indicator for childhood abuse and posttraumatic stress in youth. *Pediatrics, 129*, 410–418.

Royal College of Psychiatry. (2003). *Gender identity disorders in children and adolescents: Guidance for management*. CR63

Serbin, L., Poulin-Dubois, D., Colburne, K., Sen, M., & Eichstedt, J. (2001). Gender stereotyping in infancy: Visual preferences for and knowledge of gender-stereotyped toys in the second year. *International Journal of Behavioral Development, 25*, 7–15.

Serbin, L., Poulin-Dubois, D., & Eichstedt, J. (2002). Infants' responses to gender-inconsistent events. *Infancy, 3*, 531–542.

Shumer, D., & Spack, N. (2013). Current management of gender identity disorder in childhood and adolescence: Guidelines, barriers and areas of controversy. *Current Opinion in Endocrinology, Diabetes and Obesity, 20*, 69–73.

Steensma, T., Biemond, R., de Boer, F., & Cohen-Kettenis, P. (2011, January). Desisting and persisting gender dysphoria after childhood: A qualitative follow-up study. *Clinical Child Psychology and Psychiatry, 16*, 499–516.

Stevens, M., Golombok, S., Beveridge, M., & The ALSPAC Study Team. (2002). Does father absence influence children's gender development? Findings from a general population study of preschool children. *Parenting Science and Practice, 2*, 47–60.

Stevenson, M., & Black, K. (1988). Paternal absence and sex-role development: A meta-analysis. *Child Development, 59*, 793–814.

Stoller, R. (1968). Differential diagnoses: Transvestism and transsexualism. In J. Sutherland (Ed.), *Sex and gender* (pp. 220–226). London: Hogarth Press.

Szkrybalo, J., & Ruble, D. (1999). "God made me a girl": Sex-category constancy judgments and explanations revisited. *Developmental Psychology, 32*, 392–402.

Uddenberg, N., Walinder, J., & Hojerback, T. (1979). Parental contact in male and female transsexuals. *Acta Psychiatrica Scandinavica, 60*, 113–120.

World Professional Association for Transgender Health (WPATH). (2013). *Standards of Care. Version 7.* World Professional Association for Transgender Health. Retrieved September 2013, from http://www.wpath.org/publications_standards.cfm.

Zucker, K., Green, R., Garofano, C., Bradley, S., Williams, K., & Rebach, H. (1994). Prenatal preferences of mothers of feminine and masculine boys. *Journal of Abnormal Child Psychology, 22*, 1–13.

9

Adolescence, Young Adulthood, and Transsexualism–Transgenderism

9.0 INTRODUCTION

Adolescence and young adulthood is a period filled with many changes for transsexual and transgender people. Knowledge of physiological, learning, and social phenomena that occur in adolescence and the young adult period are important for understanding transsexualism and transgenderism (TSTG). Physiological changes that accompany puberty can cause panic among transsexual and transgender teens due to irreversible changes that conflict with their congruent gender behavior category but puberty blocking can help.

Learning phenomena include gender behavior learning and sexual arousal learning. This is the time when gender behavior matures. This is the time when sexual arousal becomes associated with stimuli and is learned based on increased spontaneous sexual arousal and novelty; sexual arousal is learned through classical conditioning and can therefore be extinguished.

Social phenomena include increased rejection and implementation of strategies to reduce it. Although families and cultures may tolerate TSTG in children, intolerance increases steeply for overt teen and adult transsexual and transgender behavior during this period. Bullying and violence due to rejection at school and in public increase and become more dangerous in terms of the capability for injury by peers. Some additional transsexual and transgender people retreat into secrecy and some may discontinue TSTG behavior. As discussed in this chapter and in Chapter 12, the fact that sexual arousal can be extinguished eliminates fetishism as a mechanism in TSTG. Some transsexual and transgender people flee their circumstances into distracting risky occupations such as the military. Flight into marriage in the belief that these can "cure" TSTG is also common.

9.1 PUBERTY AND PUBERTY BLOCKING

The start of puberty in adolescence can disrupt TSTG social transition begun in childhood by inducing irreversible unwanted body changes and increased urgency for transsexual transition. Although some transsexual and transgender individuals opt for blocking hormones prior to the onset of puberty, typically they do not start blockers until early signs of puberty actual begin. Depending when blockers start, many of the unwanted signs of puberty are reduced for transsexual and transgender teens. Full breast development can be avoided for female-to-male (FTM), and voice change can be avoided for male-to-female (MTF). For FTM, blocking should be started at or before Tanner Stage 2 of breast development (Hembree, 2011) according to the Endocrine Society (Hembree, 2011) and World Professional Association for Transgender Health (WPATH) guidelines (2013).

De Vries, Steensma, Doreleijers, and Cohen-Kettenis (2011) found that adolescents using blockers had fewer emotional problems and depression decreased for both male-to-female (MTF) and female-to-male (FTM) transsexuals aged 12 to 16. In this study, all 70 participants completed puberty blocking, and all continued into cross-sex hormone transsexual hormone therapy transition.

For those taking blockers, the decision to start cross-sex hormones for transsexual transition is typically made at age 16 to 18 (Cohen-Kettenis, Delemarre-van de Waal, & Gooren, 2008), depending on the protocol in use and the individual. The decision to start cross-sex hormones requires consultation with family and guardians. Once the individual starts transsexual transition, guidelines (WPATH, 2013) are followed for initial hormone therapy (HT) decision and subsequent treatment. More detailed information on puberty blocking is included in Section 8.4.2.

9.2 GENDER TASK LEARNING

During adolescence and early adulthood, people are expected by their cultures to learn the gender behaviors or tasks of their assigned gender behavior category. During childhood, they become familiar with such tasks, but start to practice and perfect them during adolescence and young adulthood. A taxonomy of gender tasks is useful for characterizing the gender behavior categories of a culture (Bevan, 2011). Psychologists use similar taxonomies to define user tasks to develop training requirements, systems, and workloads for various categories of users (McNeese & Vidulich, 2002). In a binary masculine-feminine gender system, some behavior tasks will be clearly classified to one or the other gender, and some will be in between. It is the overall pattern of task performances that will determine how people in that culture will perceive the gender behavior category that the person is following.

Because of secrecy, many transsexual and transgender people are forced to learn gender behaviors belonging to an incongruent gender behavior category. They spend less time practicing the gender behaviors belonging to their congruent gender behavior category. Consequently when transsexuals and transgender people come out, they have much remedial learning to do to be perceived as authentic. The remedial work comes at a time when some may be going through a second puberty due to HT. The MTF "glam" look suitable for going out to bars and nightclubs is not suitable for day-to-day living. More authentic looks have to be learned. Wig maintenance becomes less important than learning to blow-dry real hair. At first, many out transsexuals and transgender people will have awkward appearances until they adapt. This makes them less able to pass and more vulnerable to rejection.

9.3 SEXUAL AROUSAL LEARNING AND TSTG

Knowledge of the scientific findings concerning sexual arousal is important to understanding that TSTG is not a form of fetish behavior. Transgender people are more interested in the relaxation and relief that cross-dressing brings than in sexual arousal (Buhrich, 1978). Although transsexual and transgender people may initially get sexually aroused while cross-dressing and cross-presenting, this sexual arousal does not persist. TSTG persists long after the sexual arousal fades. Sexual arousal is learned, and although it starts to be learned in childhood, the learning becomes more intensive during adolescence due to hormones that sensitize sex organs and influence sexual arousal.

Sexual arousal obeys the laws of **classical** or **Pavlovian conditioning**, which has been demonstrated in both male (Hoffman, Janssen, & Turner, 2004; Janssen, Everaerd, Spiering, & Janssen, 2010; Lalumière & Quinsey, 1998;) and female (Both, Spiering, Laan, Belcome, van den Heuvel, & Everaerd, 2008; Both, Brauer, & Laan 2011; Hoffman, 2012; Hoffman, Janssen, & Turner, 2004) humans. This is supported by similar studies in animals (Köksal et al., 2004).

Classical or Pavlovian conditioning involves a paradigm in which a neutral stimulus precedes a physiological response. In the typical experimental design of Pavlov, meat powder was presented to a dog, which would salivate in anticipation of eating the food. The meat powder was called the **unconditioned**

stimulus because it reliably produced salivation, the **unconditioned response**. He would then ring a bell before presenting the meat powder. After several trials, the sound of the bell would also trigger salivation. The sound of the bell was termed the **conditioned stimulus**, and the resulting salivation was termed the **conditioned response**.

So it is with sexual arousal, only in this case the unconditioned stimulus is a stimulus that reliably produces a sexual arousal response. The unconditioned stimulus could result from friction due to masturbation, although in adolescence it could also occur from friction of clothing or romantic touching because sex organs become sensitized due to hormone surges. The unconditioned stimulus could also result from previous conditioning experiences during romantic relationships. The neural system controlling romantic relationships or pair-bonding appears to be separate from sexual arousal, involves other hormones, and appears to be more related to sexual orientation.

To complete the classical conditioning paradigm, the conditioned stimulus could be, for example, lipstick, leather clothing, or lace. All unconditioned stimuli are not the same. In particular, novel stimuli are easier to condition because they gain attention and provoke physiological responses (Ford & Beach, 1952). Novel stimuli like body modifications, piercings or motorcycle clothing, feminine perfume, or even mild pain can gain attention. The unconditioned response is, of course, sexual arousal.

There are several principles of classical conditioning, and two are particularly important to an understanding of TSTG. We described the first principle earlier, that of **acquisition**. The strength of the resulting learned conditioned response varies with the number of exposures and novelty of the unconditioned stimulus. The second principle is extinction. **Extinction** refers to a change in the parading in which the conditioned stimulus is presented, but the unconditioned stimulus is no longer presented. With repeated trials, the conditioned response no longer appears, and the unconditioned stimulus is no longer effective. The link between the conditioned stimulus and the conditioned response is no longer effective.

The classical conditioning of sexual arousal is mediated by unconscious functions and does not require conscious thought or control, although conscious perception certainly occurs afterward in humans. This means that sexual arousal conditioning is independent from gender behavior categories and sexual orientation. Sexual arousal conditioning follows erotic experience in whatever direction it leads. So, for example, leather clothing could be an arousing stimulus (conditioned stimulus) whether male–female, feminine–masculine gender, or straight–gay sexual orientation. Novelty of the conditioned stimulus is also judged by these unconscious mechanisms and is not under conscious control.

Many nonprofessionals and some mental health professionals (see Section 12.1.1) explicitly or implicitly believe that TSTG is due to the pleasurable effects of sexual arousal to clothes or other aspects of presentation in the gender behavior category not culturally assigned to the TSTG. No doubt transsexuals and transgender people do get sexually aroused when their cross-dressing starts but the classical conditioning principle of extinction indicates that increased exposure will result in reduced sexual arousal. TSTG behavior continues long after extinction has taken place, indicating that sexual arousal is not a causal factor in TSTG.

Cross-dressing is the perfect opportunity for extinction of sexual arousal. Many conditioned stimuli are presented at one time without an unconditioned stimulus. In fact, therapists use a similar strategy to desensitize or extinguish emotions such as phobias and anxiety, which they call **flooding desensitization** (Levis & Castelda, 2007). It also occurs in everyday life when a child enters a new school full of previously unencountered stimuli or when someone starts a new job. After experiencing school or a new workplace for several months, emotional responses are reduced or extinguished.

Transsexual and transgender people are forced to learn an incongruent gender behavior category as well as surreptitiously scrutinize people in their congruent gender behavior category to learn by observation and modeling. This means that because transsexuals and transgender people pay particular attention to the details of cross-sex dressing or presentation, they may be more vulnerable to sexual arousal conditioning. They are also expected to learn about sexual behavior. Transsexual and transgender people may become sexually aroused by such detailed observation and learning about their congruent gender behavior category.

This understanding of sexual arousal conditioning also helps explain why "early blooming" transsexuals tend to be classified as homosexual transsexuals, whereas "later blooming" transsexuals tend to be classified as heterosexual. The late bloomers are usually those who come out after living in secrecy while trying to pretend they are not transsexual or transgender. During childhood, adolescence, and young adulthood, transsexual and transgender homosexuals may form pair bonds and have romantic encounters with same-sex individuals, whereas the late bloomers form these bonds and sexual arousal linkages with opposite-sex people. The late bloomers have lots of learned opposite-sex linkages that may complicate the pursuit of their congruent gender behavior category by causing unwanted sexual arousal. Transsexuals may show a characteristic response of opposite-sex arousal, which persists into the postoperative transition period (Lawrence, Latty, Chivers, & Bailey, 2005). However, these late bloomers eventually fall in line with the tendency of most postoperative transsexuals to form sexual relationships with same-sex individuals (see Section 12.5). The interaction of pair bonding and sexual arousal conditioning deserves additional study.

All children going through puberty experience growth and increased sensation due to hormone flows that results in frequent sexual arousal. The sexual arousal may be due to romantic encounters, exposure to novel stimuli, or masturbation, or may simply occur spontaneously. Sexual arousal can be acquired and can be extinguished according to classical conditioning rules. This means that TSTG cannot be due to a fetish because it persists beyond extinction of sexual arousal for opposite gender stimuli (Prince, 1976). Indeed, surveys of MTF TSTG in support groups report that TSTG do not cross-dress for sexual arousal but instead for relaxation and relieving masculine demands (Buhrich, 1978).

9.4 FAMILY AND CULTURAL REJECTION

It is during this period that family and cultural rejection of TSTG behavior becomes most intense. Childhood transgressions against culture can be overlooked and tolerated due to the commonly held belief that children will "grow out of it." But during adolescence, TSTG behavior may become more obvious and overt. Family rejection of TSTG behavior is supported by cultural institutions such as churches and communities that advocate intolerance and, in turn, reject parents and families if they tolerate TSTG behavior.

Studies show that positive emotional relations in adolescence are vital to the mental health of transsexuals and transgender people (Ryan, Russell, Huebner, Diaz, & Sanchez, 2010). However, TSTG behavior sometimes results in the absence of warm and intense contact in cross-sex parents and poor emotional relations with the same-sex parent (Uddenberg, Walinder, Hojerback, & Cohen-Kettenis, 1979).

Family rejection for many transsexuals and transgender people means becoming homeless without the skills to support themselves. Many turn to street crime to survive. Because of cultural rejection, many government institutions are not allowed to provide needed assistance, even though street crimes such as drugs and prostitution represent a significant public health threat (see Section 2.2).

A few transsexuals and transgender people try to continue their public presentation in their congruent gender behavior category, but they are subject to cultural and family rejection. FTM can express themselves more freely, but nonetheless only 33% of FTM can present in androgynous or masculine style as a "tomboy." Only 2% express their TSTG (Kennedy, 2008, 2010).

9.5 BULLYING AND VIOLENCE

Transsexual or transgender people are subject to the threat of bullying and violence by their peers or others, which may be encouraged by culture (see Section 2.4). More than 60% of TSTG adolescents experience violent attacks (Moran & Sharpe, 2004). Potential bullies pay particular attention to violations of gender behavior categories because they, too, are in the process of learning appropriate behaviors. TSTG adolescents are particularly at risk at middle and high schools (Cohen-Kettenis & van Gooren, 1999; Grossman & D'Augelli, 2006). Families and cultural organizations contribute to this violence due to their rejection of TSTG. Cultural rejection of TSTG helps sanction violence because of these violations and because they regard transsexuals and transgender people as easy prey. It is during this period when peer bullying and violence become most intense in schools and on the street.

9.6 SECRECY, DISCONTINUATION, AND ADULT OUTCOMES

As was discussed in Section 2.1, for those transsexual and transgender people who adopt a strategy of secrecy surrounding their cross-dressing, puberty intensifies the stress of keeping their secret and their loneliness. The biological changes in puberty increase this stress because typically the secret-keeping transsexuals and transgender people do not have anyone they can trust to discuss their problems. Secrecy results in a vicious cycle in which individuals deliberately isolate themselves to avoid inadvertently revealing their secret. Isolation results in fewer friends they can trust. Secrecy also results in loneliness and depression (Kelly, 2002), which undoubtedly contribute to the number of suicide attempts.

The clinical literature indicates that many transsexual and transgender people may temporarily or permanently discontinue TSTG behavior during this period because of cultural pressures. Some clinicians have observed a gradual decrease in transgender behavior during late childhood, teenage years, and early adulthood (Wallien & Cohen-Kettenis, 2008) when cultural pressures to conform intensify. However, it is likely that many transsexual and transgender adolescents just go into hiding to express their TSTG behavior. Longitudinal studies of the TSTG population are scarce but, in clinical studies, many individuals who were overtly transgender in childhood report that discontinuation of their TSTG behavior starts at age 10 to 12 years (Steensma, Biemond, and de Boer, 2011) and increases until early adulthood. At age 10 to 12, family and cultural pressure start to force discontinuation. These studies also do not reveal how many TSTG adopt secrecy in childhood and continue into adolescence.

Many clinical investigators believe that childhood transgender behavior is associated with adult outcomes of non-TSTG homosexuality and transsexualism (Bailey & Zucker, 1995; Davenport, 1986; Drummond, Bradley, Peterson-Badali, & Zucker 2008; Green, 1979; Rieger, Linsenmeier, Gygax, & Bailey, 2008; Whitam, 1980; Zuger, 1966, 1984, 1988). However, the most recent study indicates that the proportion of transgender children who become non-TSTG homosexuals is relatively small. Steensma, Biemond, & de Baer (2011) found that only 10.2% to 12.2% become non-TSTG homosexuals. This may not be statistically significantly different from the frequency of homosexuality in the population once biases in the clinical sample are removed.

It is clear that many TSTG emerge from secrecy later in life. Some remain as closeted cross-dressers into advanced ages. We do not have good longitudinal studies on these secretive TSTG because most of them never perceive the need to see a mental health professional.

9.7 FLIGHT TO RISKY OCCUPATIONS AND MARRIAGE

Some TSTG enter high-risk occupations or get married in an attempt to "cure" themselves. High-risk occupations such as the military, firefighting, or police work keep TSTG involved in problems outside of themselves, but TSTG frequently reemerges. Many find that their marriages fail, due in part to the reemergence of TSTG behavior.

Dr. George Brown was an M.D. who served in the U.S. Air Force and now in the Veterans Administration. He published his first paper on MTF TSTG military flight in 1988. As a follow-up in the Veterans Affairs Administration, he and his colleagues published a paper (Blosnich et al., 2013) indicating that TSTG are twice as likely to join the military. The subjects were a sample of 5 million exiting servicemen. This study indicates that TSTG are overrepresented in the military when compared with the general population. In the military, they cannot currently receive treatment for problems resulting from TSTG, and coming out is grounds for discharge. See Section 2.10 for a discussion of the status of the movement to allow TSTG to serve in the military.

Brown's interpretation is that transsexual and transgender servicemen join to exhibit hypermasculinity. This is supported by quotes from transsexual and transgender people that they joined the service "to become a real man." Other interpretations are possible, including the notion that TSTG want to get absorbed in activities that are socially valued and are a distraction from their TSTG motivation. Transsexual and transgender people may also engage in such activities to support their concealment strategy because few people would suspect them of being TSTG in such vocations or avocations (Kennedy, 2010).

There are also anecdotal reports that TSTG are overrepresented in such risky professions as firefighting and police work or risky avocations such as skydiving, but there is no scientific data on this issue.

A phenomena known as "marriage flight," in which transsexual and transgender people, usually MTF, get married to be "cured," has also been reported. In reported dialogues, they have come to believe that if they get married and have regular sex that the TSTG will disappear. Nothing could be further from the truth. Marriage does not "cure" TSTG, and frequently the emergence of TSTG causes family difficulties and divorce. Because of this, TSTG support groups typically have programs for significant others (SOs) to help them deal with their partner's TSTG. After the transsexual or transgender spouse comes out, the SO may feel deceived and believe that the partner's TSTG is somehow due to his or her own sexual inadequacy.

Things are particularly difficult for the SOs of transsexuals. Although the law has been changed in many localities, some countries still require divorce before a transsexual can complete transition. Increasingly, however, transsexuals and their partners stay together after transition even though they have to deal with many practical problems.

9.8 SUMMARY

Knowledge of physiological, learning, and social phenomena that occur in adolescence and the young adult period are important for understanding TSTG. These include puberty and puberty blocking, learning gender tasks, family and cultural rejection, bullying and violence, secrecy and discontinuation, and flight from TSTG to risky occupations or marriage.

REFERENCES

Bailey, M., & Zucker, K. (1995). Childhood sex-typed behavior and sexual orientation: A conceptual analysis and quantitative review. *Developmental Psychology, 31*, 43–55.

Bevan, T. (2011, September). *Biopsychology of transsexualism and transgenderism*. World Professional Association for Transgender Health Symposium, Atlanta, GA.

Blosnich, J., Brown, G., Shipherd, J., Kauth, M., Plegari, M., & Bossarte, R. (2013). Prevalence of gender identity disorder and suicide risk among transgender veterans utilizing veterans' health administration care. *American Journal of Public Health, 103*, e27–32.

Both, S., Brauer, M., & Laan, E. (2011, November). Classical conditioning of sexual response in women: A replication study. *Journal of Sexual Medicine, 8*, 3116–3131.

Both, S., Spiering, M., Laan, E., Belcome, S., van den Heuvel, B., & Everaerd, W. (2008). Unconscious classical conditioning of sexual arousal: Evidence for the conditioning of female genital arousal to subliminally presented sexual stimuli. *Journal of Sexual Medicine, 5*, 100–109.

Brown, G. (1988). Transsexuals in the military: Flight into hypermasculinity. *Archives of Sexual Behavior, 17*, 527–537.

Buhrich, N. (1978). Motivation for cross-dressing in heterosexual transvestism. *Acta Psychiatrica Scandinavica, 57*, 145–152.

Cohen-Kettenis, P., Delemarre-van de Waal, H., & Gooren, L. (2008). The treatment of adolescent transsexuals: Changing insights. *Journal of Sexual Medicine, 5*, 1892–1897.

Cohen-Kettenis, P., & van Gooren, L. (1999). Transsexualism: A review of etiology, diagnosis and treatment. *Journal of Psychosomatic Research, 46*, 315–333.

Davenport, C. (1986). A follow-up study of 10 feminine boys. *Archives of Sexual Behavior, 15*, 511–517.

De Vries, L. C., Steensma, T. D., Doreleijers, T. A., Cohen-Kettenis, P. T. (2011). Puberty suppression in adolescents with gender identity disorder: A prospective follow up study. *Journal of Sexual Education, 8*, 2276–2283.

Drummond, K., Bradley, S., Peterson-Badali, M., & Zucker, K. (2008). A follow-up study of girls with gender identity disorder. *Developmental Psychology, 44*, 34–45.

Ford, C., & Beach, F. (1952). *Patterns of sexual behavior*. New York: Harper.

Green, R. (1979). Childhood cross-gender behavior and subsequent sexual preference. *American Journal of Psychiatry, 136*, 106–108.

Grossman, A. H., & D'Augelli, A. R. (2006). Transgender youth: Invisible and vulnerable. *Journal of Homosexuality, 51*, 111–128.

Hembree, W. (2011). Guidelines for pubertal suspension and gender reassignment for transgender adolescents. *Child Adolescent Psychiatric Clinics of North America, 20*, 725–732.

Hoffman, H. (2012, February). Considering the role of conditioning in sexual orientation. *Archives of Sexual Behavior, 41*, 63–71.

Hoffman, H., Janssen, E., & Turner, S. (2004). Classical conditioning of sexual arousal in women and men: Effects of varying awareness and biological relevance of the conditioned stimulus. *Archives of Sexual Behavior, 33*, 43–53.

Janssen, E., Everaerd, W., Spiering, M., & Janssen, J. (2010). Automatic processes and the appraisal of sexual stimuli: Toward an information processing model of sexual arousal. *Journal of Sexual Research, 37*, 8–23.

Kelly, A. (2002). *The psychology of secrets*. New York: Plenum.

Kennedy, N. (2008). Transgendered children in schools: A critical review of homophobic bullying. Safe to learn—embedding anti-bullying work in schools. *Forum, 50*, 383–396.

Kennedy, N. (2010). Transgender children: More than a theoretical challenge. *Graduate Journal of Social Science, 7*, 25–42.

Köksal, F., Domjan, M., Kurt, A., Özlem, S., Örung, S., Bowers, R., & Kumru, G. (2004). An animal model of fetishism. *Behaviour Research Therapy, 42*, 1421–1434.

Lalumière, M., & Quinsey, V. (1998). Pavlovian conditioning of sexual interests in human males. *Archives of Sexual Behavior, 27*, 241–252.

Lawrence, A., Latty, E., Chivers, M., & Bailey, J. (2005). Measurement of sexual arousal in postoperative male-to-female transsexuals using vaginal photoplethysmography. *Archives of Sexual Behavior, 34*, 135–145.

Levis, D., & Castelda, B. (2007). Stampfl's therapist directed implosive (flooding) therapy. In M. Hersen & J. Rosqvist (Eds.), *Encyclopedia of behavior modification and cognitive behavior therapy.* Thousand Oaks, CA: Sage.

McNeese, M., & Vidulich, M. (2002). *Cognitive systems engineering in military aviation environments: Avoiding cogminutia fragmentosa!* Dayton, OH: Human Systems Information Center, Wright-Patterson AFB.

Moran, L., & Sharpe, A. (2004). Violence, identity and policing: The case of violence against transgender people. *Criminal Justice, 4*, 395–417.

Prince, V. (1976). *Understanding cross-dressing.* Los Angeles: Chevalier.

Rieger, G., Linsenmeier, J., Gygax, L., & Bailey, J. (2008). Sexual orientation and childhood gender nonconformity: Evidence from home videos. *Developmental Psychology, 44*, 46–58.

Ryan, C., Russell, S. T., Huebner, D., Diaz, R., & Sanchez, J. (2010). Family acceptance in adolescence and the health of LGBT young adults. *Journal of Child Adolescent Psychiatric Nursing, 23*, 205–213.

Steensma, T., Biemond, T., & de Boer, F. (2011). Desisting and persisting gender dysphoria after childhood: A qualitative follow-up study. *Clinical Child Psychology and Psychiatry, 16*, 499–516.

Uddenberg, N., Walinder, J., Hojerback, T., & Cohen-Kettenis, P. (1979). Parental contact in male and female transsexuals. *Acta Psychiatrica Scandinavica, 60*, 113–120.

Wallien, M., & Cohen-Kettenis, P. (2008). Psychosexual outcome of gender-dysphoric children. *Journal of the American Academy of Adolescent Psychiatry, 47*, 1413–1423.

Whitam, F. (1980). The prehomosexual male child in three societies: The United States, Guatemala, and Brazil. *Archives of Sexual Behavior, 9*, 87–99.

World Professional Association for Transgender Health (WPATH). (2013). *Standards of Care. Version 7.* World Professional Association for Transgender Health. Retrieved September 2013 from http://www.wpath.org/publications_standards.cfm.

Zuger, B. (1984). Early effeminate behavior in boys. Outcome and significance for homosexuality. *Journal of Nervous and Mental Disease, 172*, 90–97.

Zuger, B. (1966). Effeminate behavior present in boys from early childhood. *Journal of Pediatrics*, 1098–1107

Zuger, B. (1988). Is early effeminate behavior in boys early homosexuality? *Comprehensive Psychiatry, 29*, 509–519.

10

Neuroanatomy and Neurophysiology

10.0 INTRODUCTION

As soon as it became apparent that transsexualism and transgenderism (TSTG) might be a biological phenomenon, researchers began to search for brain structures or functions that were different in transsexuals versus non-transsexuals. Transsexuals were used because they were believed to have the strongest motivation for TSTG. Some investigators chose to search in locations with known **sexual dimorphic brain structures** that vary with sex. *Dimorphic* simply means that the structures have a different male and a female shape, structure, size, or a combination of these. Some investigators, using magnetic resonance imaging (MRI) scanners, chose to investigate the whole brain at once. So far, all of the research has been done on transsexuals and none on nontranssexual transgender people because the investigators wanted to start with what they perceived as the extremes of TSTG.

As a starting point, some researchers searched where there were known differences between male and female neuroanatomy, for example, hypothalamic cell nucleus sizes. Such hypothalamic structures are known to have connections to sensory information and sexual reflexes in the male penis and female vagina (Bancila et al., 2002; Gelez et al., 2010). The investigators reasoned that structure and function of transsexual might correlate with the opposite birth sex. This was also a matter of practicality because nontranssexual human cadaver brain specimens are easier to acquire than transsexual brains. So it was more convenient to look first for sex differences, then for transsexual versus nontranssexual differences. The search was, in part, directed toward parts of the brain that were believed to be organized by pre-natal testosterone because there are male-female differences in these struc-tures, and if sex/aggression was organized in these locations in animals, then gender predisposition might also be organized there as well. This strategy was undoubtedly influenced by the organization-activation theories of the 1970s for sex and aggression. As we have seen, there is evidence that sex/aggression and TSTG behavior have independent mechanisms (Chapter 6).

Historically the search was directed at individual parts of the brain, but now we have the means to study brain structure and activity patterns of the entire human brain using MRI, functional MRI (fMRI), and other scanning technologies. Neuroanatomical structure and brain function are complicated, so it is necessary to know both the neuroanatomical correlates of individual structures and how those structures interact to produce behavior.

This chapter presents the known neuroanatomical correlates of TSTG including the results of investigation of individual structures as well as whole brain scanning. Because of initial strategies targeting sexual dimorphic brain structures, there are many brain structures that have not been examined for neuroanatomical correlates of TSTG.

10.1 NEUROANATOMICAL CORRELATES

10.1.1 Bed Nucleus of the Stria Terminalis

Perhaps the most often cited neuroanatomical correlate of TSTG in the lit-erature is the size and composition of a portion of the **bed nucleus of the stria terminalis** (BNST) in humans. This cell nucleus is found in the **anterior hypothalamus** near the midline of the brain (see Figure 10.1). This figure shows a head-on (coronal) cross-section of the brain near the **optic chiasm**. The optic chiasm is where the two visual nerves meet to share information, which is transmitted to the rest of the brain by the optic tracts. This figure shows the location of the BNST as well as other brain structures described below. If you put your tongue on the roof of your mouth, it will be only a few centimeters below the hypothalamus and optic chiasm.

The hypothalamus is one of the oldest structures, and it is believed to control both the autonomic nervous system and the pituitary. The autonomic nervous system controls phenomena such as heart rate, body temperature, hunger, thirst, stomach acidity, penile erection, and vaginal lubrication. The pituitary is beneath the hypothalamus, even closer to your tongue. It is responsible for secreting hor-mones into the blood stream including the sex hormones. The hypothalamus senses body chemicals and states and adjusts pituitary secretions accordingly. The anterior hypothalamus contains several sexual dimorphic structures.

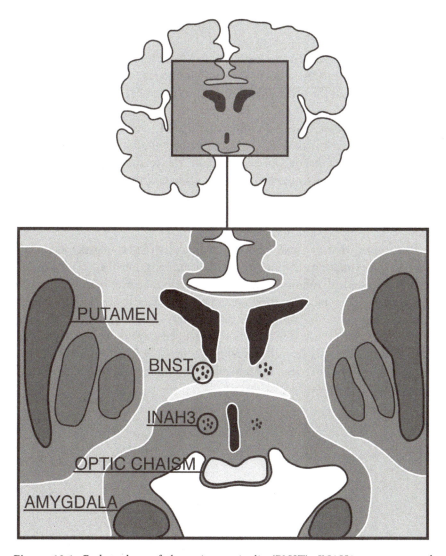

Figure 10.1. Bed nucleus of the stria terminalis (BNST), INAH3, putamen, and surrounding brain structures

The BNST is one of the sexual dimorphic structures in the anterior hypothalamus. The BNST consists of the cell bodies of neurons that connect several important structures in the brain. A neuron is a key cell in the nervous system because it processes information and transmits it to other neurons. Structures of the neuron include the cell body, dendrites that receive information from other cells, and axons that transmit the processed information to the dendrites of other cells. The cell body performs all of the usual support functions that any cell must do but in addition it supports information processing. Axons form into bundles with similar destinations, which appear white because the neurons have an outer layer of fat to improve transmission. In contrast, cell bodies appear gray.

The BNST is embedded in a group of fiber bundles that includes the anterior commissure and the stria terminalis. The anterior commissure connects structures between the two halves of the brain. The BNST provides cell bodies for the stria terminalis bundles. Fiber bundles are the "transmission lines" between structures and are extensions of cell bodies such as are found in the BNST. The stria terminalis is a relatively old fiber bundle. The stria terminalis connects with the amygdala in a spiral path. The tortuous spiral path of the stria terminalis is due to the evolutionary growth of the cerebral cortex that "pushed" several structures in a spiral path as shown in Figure 10.2. The fact that the stria terminalis persisted over evolution indicates that it must have evolutionary important functions.

It is known that the BNST provides connectivity between the amygdala and the **hypothalamus** through the stria terminalis, but the BNST also has connections with an important structure down in the lower brain stem called the ventral tegmental dopamine area. The **amygdala** is an almond-shaped structure (*amygdala* is "almond" in Latin) that is believed to mediate emotional learning and behavior from the diverse sensory inputs it receives both directly and indirectly from the cerebral cortex. The BNST supplies the cell bodies that connect between the amygdala and the hypothalamus through a fiber bundle known as the stria terminalis.

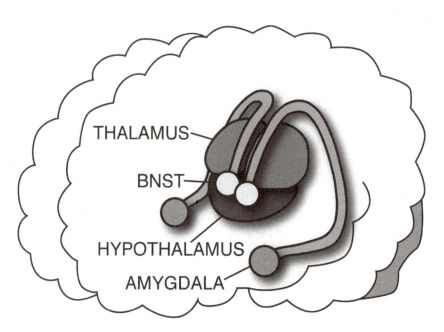

Figure 10.2. Bed nucleus of the stria terminalis (BNST) connection to amygdala

The BNST also connects with the ventral tegmental area that supplies dopamine to forebrain structures. **Dopamine** is a neurotransmitter that chemically transmits information from one neuron to another (usually axon to dendrite). Dopamine release is associated with reward, pleasure, and addiction. Drugs such as cocaine, amphetamines, and nicotine cause release and intensification of dopamine effects. The BNST through the ventral tegmental area are thus functionally positioned to have an important impact on behavior.

The BNST is clearly involved in primitive emotions as indicated by animal experiments on noncontact penile erection, fear and anxiety, startle reflex, and learning under stress. The BNST is influenced by testosterone levels and, in fact, concentrates testosterone in some of its cells. Testosterone crosses the blood-brain barrier and is converted by the **aromatase enzyme** or catalyst to estradiol that causes male organization in the BNST and other structures. A division of the BNST was shown by Guillamón, Segovia, and del Abril (1998) and Allen and Gorski (2004) to be approximately 2.5 times larger in human males than females.

An often-cited BNST study (Zhou, Hofman, Gooren, & Swaab, 1995) found that for a group of seven MTF transsexuals, the BNST was found to be smaller than both male and female but closer to the BNST structures of control females. The study defined the volume of the BNST by locating vasoactive intestinal peptide (VIP) innervation of the nucleus. VIP is involved in a variety of functions, one of which is a timekeeping function in the nearby hypothalamus suprachiasmatic nucleus (SCN), which communicates with a similar function in the BNST (Amir, Waddington, Robinson, & Stewart, 2004; Zhou, Hofman, & Swaab, 1995). Some of the transsexuals included in the Zhou study were also participants in a study of detection of **somatostatin**-containing cells in the BNST. Somatostatin is a peptide that is manufactured in hypothalamic structures. Similar results were obtained for numbers of neurons (Kruijver et al., 2000) in the BNST.

Some took these results as support for the idea that TSTG is a biological phenomenon, but others began to criticize the study. The first criticism was that the sample size of transsexual brains was too small. No doubt it would be highly desirable to have more than seven donated postmortem transsexual brains, but that was the available sample in the Netherlands at the time. In defense of the sample size, analysis did show statistical significance.

The second criticism lodged against this study was that the transsexuals had been taking hormones that might reduce the size of structures sensitive to testosterone levels. This criticism was made despite the fact that one transsexual had ceased taking hormones 15 months before her death. The size of her BNST was in the same range as the other transsexuals. Of course, the results for this single "control" transsexual cannot to be used to rule out permanent (greater than 15 months) changes of hormone therapy (HT).

An MRI study by Pol et al. (2006) has been cited in criticism of the BNST study. This MRI study involved comparison of in vivo MRI scans of MTF transsexuals before they started HT to rescans taken 6 months into HT. Indeed, the results of this MRI were dramatic, with the shrinkage of the hypothalamus and neighboring regions and an average overall reduction in brain size of 30 cc. However, the MRI did not indicate that the BNST was involved in this shrinkage. The MRI that was used did not have sufficient resolution to recognize and measure a structure as small as the BNST, and tissue shrinkage can move structures away from their usual locations.

The third criticism raised about this study was that the BNST does not mature until late teens/early adulthood (Chung, De Vries, & Swaab, 2002), whereas realization of TSTG occurs in childhood. During early postnatal development, neurons in the brain proliferate, and those that are not used gradually undergo **apoptosis**, or programmed cell death, otherwise characterized as "use it or lose it." Divergence between male and female BNST volume begins around age 14. The number of cells in the BNST is stable or somewhat declines after age 18 to 19. Although it is true that the BNST matures at a different age from TSTG realization, BNST neurons must be functioning throughout childhood and adolescence; otherwise they would be eliminated by apoptosis.

It appears that the size and composition of the BNST correlates with TSTG, despite the criticisms raised against the correlation.

10.1.2 INAH3 Nucleus

The potential association of the **INAH3 hypothalamic nucleus** with TSTG was the subject of research by Garcia-Falgueras and Swaab (2008) based on previous discoveries that the nucleus was larger in males than females in postmortem histology (Allen, Hines, Shryne, & Gorski, 1989; Byne et al., 2001). This small nucleus (Figure 10-1) is located at the base of the anterior hypothalamus (below the BNST) and was named accordingly as the interstitial nucleus of the anterior hypothalamus (INAH). There are four such nuclei, but the nucleus designated INAH3 is consistently larger in males than females. In humans, little is known about the INAH3, but it is believed to be part of the sexually dimorphic anterior hypothalamus that is involved in sex reflex circuits and maternal behavior in animals. Several postmortem studies show that the INAH3 is sexually dimorphic. Allen, Hines, Shryne, & Gorski (1989) found that both the INAH3 and the neighboring INAH2 were on the average 2.8 times larger in males than females, but that the INAH2 size varied with hormone levels. Byne et al. (2001) confirmed this result but did not find any size difference in the other three neighboring nuclei (INAH1, 3, 4). LeVay (1991) found that INAH3 size was similar in size to females in homosexual males, and subsequently Byne et al. (2001) found that homosexual males had INAH3 that was similar to heterosexual females but the number of cells was reduced.

Garcia-Falgueras and Swaab (2008) found that MTF transsexuals had cell size and numbers similar to females. They also found that the INAH3 was 1.9 times larger in males than females and in the male also contained 2.3 times the number of cells. The six postmortem male-to-female (MTF) transsexuals included in the study had size and numbers similar to females. Eight of the MTF transsexuals had been castrated, and all were taking estrogen at death. The one female-to-male (FTM) transsexuals had volume and numbers similar to males, even though his testosterone treatment had been suspended before death. The authors believed that the INAH3 might be a marker and part of a complex network for TSTG. Garcia-Falgueras and Swaab (2008) interpreted these results as indicating that INAH3 size may be correlated with sexual orientation, whereas INAH3 cell numbers might be correlated with TSTG. Differences with the results of LeVay (1991) could therefore be due to histology technique and/or absence of cell counting.

10.1.3 Corpus Callosum Shape

The corpus callosum is a prominent white matter fiber structure that connects the two hemispheres, as shown in Figure 10.3. This figure shows three views of the corpus callosum. This first view (upper left) is a head-on (coronal) simplified cross-section that shows where it bridges the two hemispheres. The second (upper right) view shows a side view (sagittal view), which shows the extent of how it connects the two hemispheres. The third view (lower) shows the shape of the corpus callosum in side view. Several studies have analyzed the shape of the cross-section in this view, and two have involved TSTG subjects.

Emory, Williams, Cole, Amparo, and Meyer (1991) found in vivo MRI differences in the size of the corpus callosum (CC) in MTF and FTM transsexuals, but they were unable to quantify the differences. Later, Yakota, Kawamura, and Kameya (2005) found differences in the shape of the corpus callosum using MRI and a geometric model that analyzed shape parameters. Yakota, Kawamura, & Kameya (2005) measured differences in CC shape along a constructed shape axis between male and female. The model was shown to be 74% accurate in categorizing males versus females. The CC shapes of the MTF (n = 22) were found to be closer to females (n = 211), and the FTM (n = 28) were found to be closer to males (n = 211). These studies follow the line of evidence that the CC varies in shape dimorphically (Allen, 1991; Clarke & Zaidel, 1994; De Lacoste-Utamsing & Holloway, 1982; Steinmetz et al., 1992). The female CC tends to have larger and more bulbous shapes.

It is a matter of debate whether differences in the CC are involved in handedness. It would be important for testing of the two-factor theory of TSTG to compare CC correlates of handedness with those of TSTG. Witelson (1985) found that the CC was larger in non-right-handers, but more recently Preuss et al. (2002) and Luders et al. (2009) found no differences. Although perhaps

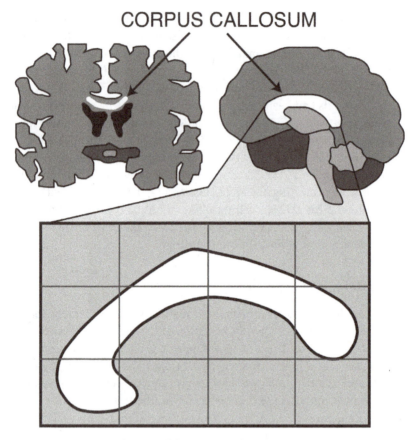

Figure 10.3. Location and views of the corpus callosum

not correlated with handedness, the CC is clearly involved in coordinating functions between hemispheres.

10.2 MRI AND FMRI

Using MRI and fMRI scanners, researchers have begun to look for structures and functions that differ between TSTG and non-TSTG. They began looking for differences in white and gray matter.

10.2.1 Gray Matter Surveys

Gray matter surveys can be conducted in full MRI brain scans. The structures that can be resolved depend on the scanner resolution. Gray matter consists mainly of neuron cell bodies, not fiber bundles as for white matter.

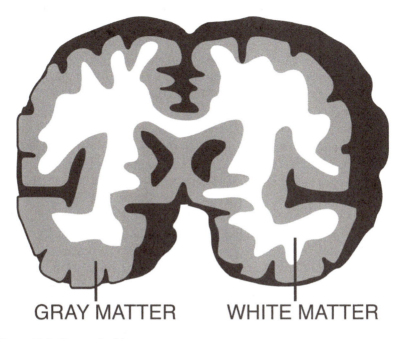

GRAY MATTER   WHITE MATTER

Figure 10.4. Gray and white matter

Luders et al. (2009) conducted the first gray matter scan to look for differences between MTF transsexuals and males/females. He found that the pattern of gray matter was similar between pre-HT MTF transsexuals and natal males except for one structure—the right putamen. (The location of the putamen is shown in Figure 10.1.) Typically, the right putamen is larger in the female than in the male. The size of this structure was larger than natal males and fell within the female range for MTF transsexuals. The right putamen mediates sensory and movement tasks for the left hand (Merchant, Zainos, Hernandez, Salinas, & Romo, 1997), so an enlarged right putamen may be an indicator of increased non-right-handedness.

10.2.2 White Matter Survey

There have been three surveys of white matter for TSTG. The term *white matter* pertains to neuron fiber bundles and structures that connect different parts of the brain (see Figure 10.4). They are white because they are layered with white fat, which increases neural transmission speed. The corpus callosum is an example of white matter (10.1.3). Gray matter consists of neuron cell bodies. All three of these studies were performed by a team working in Spain.

The first survey (Rametti et al., 2011b) looked for microstructure differences between pre-HT MTF transsexuals (*n* = 18) and non-TSTG control males (*n* = 19) and females (*n* = 19) using an MRI technique known as diffusion tensor imaging (DTI). DTI highlights the Brownian motion of water in brain structures, which is typically aligned inside fiber bundles and unaligned or *anisotropic* outside of fiber bundles. Water motion is more likely aligned or anisotropic inside fiber bundles than other parts of the brain. The white matter structure pattern of the MTF transsexuals fell between the male and female control groups for several fiber bundles, in particular, the *superior longitudinal fasciculus* (SLF), *right anterior cingulum* (RAC), *the right forceps minor* (RFM), and the *right corticospinal tract* (RCST). The SLF consists of the major fiber bundles that connect the cerebrum and cortex. The RAC wraps around the *CC* (see Section 10.1.3) and connects structures of the limbic system that are involved in mediation of emotion. The RFM is the anterior portion of the CC that connects left and right frontal lobes. The right frontal lobe is primarily nonverbal but ideates future events and emotion. The RCST sends information from the cerebral cortex to the spinal cord and is responsible for conscious motor control. The right tract controls the left hand and left side of the body. Remember that TSTG tend to be more non-right-handed and will frequently use their left hand.

The second survey involved pre-HT FTM transsexuals (Rametti et al., 2011a). This was again a DTI survey in which the direction of Brownian motion of water molecules was assessed to make fiber bundles more visible. The results of 18 FTM transsexuals were compared with 24 males and 19 females. The patterns observed for FTM TS were similar to males except for a weak difference in the *cortical spinal tract* (CST).

After 7 months of HT (Rametti et al., 2012) 15 of the FTM transsexuals were found to have significant differences in the SLF compared with their pretreatment values. The SLF consists of the major fiber bundles that connect the cerebrum and cortex and was one of the same fiber bundles shown to be different from male controls to pre-HT MTF (Rametti et al., 2012). The results of this study show that the effects of testosterone HT resulted in changes to the cortical fiber connections but not to fiber bundles elsewhere in the brain.

These DTI MRI scanning studies are the first step in understanding the structures involved in TSTG. How these structures work together with the rest of the brain with potential TSTG involvement remains to be seen.

10.2.3 fMRI

Much fMRI research has focused on sex differences in brain structure activation during various tasks, but three studies have found differences between transsexuals versus nontranssexuals. Most fMRI detect activation in brain structures through increases in iron content due to increased blood flow to the activated structures.

Both Bell, Willson, Wilman, Dave, and Silverstone (2006) and Gizewski, Krause, Wanke, Forsting, and Senf (2006) found sex differences in fMRI activation during various mental tasks including mental rotation, spatial attention, and word-generation tasks.

Later, Schöning et al. (2010) conducted the first fMRI in vivo experiments involving MTF transsexuals and found differences in the **cerebral cortex**, the outer layer of the brain involved in higher functions. Three transsexual groups were compared on a mental rotation task for fMRI activation: a pre-HT group, a MTF transsexual group that had started HT, and a control male group. Both transsexual groups showed increased activation of the occipital regions and decreased activation of the left parietal cortex compared with the control male group. There were no differences between the MTF transsexual groups, indicating that there was no effect of the HT on this task. The task used typically involves the left parietal cortex in Brodmann areas 7A and 7B, generally involved in locating objects in space. The increased activation of the occipital regions in the transsexual groups would indicate additional visual processing of the stimuli as to shape.

Gizewski et al. (2009) tested groups of 12 pre-HT MTF transsexuals, males and females, on their activation patterns during exposure to erotic visual materials. The males showed specific activation in the thalamus, amygdala, orbital cortex, and insular cortex, but the MTF, transsexuals and the females did not. This result might be interpreted in terms of classical conditioning of sexual arousal theory to mean that the MTF transsexuals and females were desensitized to the erotic visual stimuli.

Ku et al. (2013) found increases in functional organization between transsexuals and nontranssexuals for both MTF and FTM. They found that there were functional circuits involving the ventral tegmental area, the anterior cingulate, and genital representation. This study used fMRI in conjunction with visual material depicting both erotic and nonerotic activities.

Using the putative sex pheromones AND and EST, Berglund, Lindstrom, Dhejne-Helmy, and Savic (2008) found that nonhomosexual MTF transsexuals showed activation to both pheromones, whereas males showed hypothalamic activation to EST and females to AND. (AND is a testosterone derivative 4,16-androstadian-3-one from male sweat, and EST is an estrogen-like compound 1, 3, 5, (10), 16-tetraen-3-ol found in female urine.) In this study, it was important to identify sexual orientation because differences have been observed for homosexual males for these compounds (Savic, Berglund, & Lindstrom, 2005).

10.3 SUMMARY

Neuroanatomical and neurophysiological differences exist between transsexuals and nontranssexuals, supporting the idea that TSTG has a biological basis. These differences are found in many places in the brain, indicating that the structures mediating gender predisposition may not have a single location but are distributed throughout the brain.

REFERENCES

Allen, L., & Gorski, R. (2004). Sex difference in the bed nucleus of the stria terminalis of the human brain. *Journal of Comprehensive Neurology, 302,* 697–706.

Allen, L., Hines, M., Shryne, J., & Gorski, A. (1989). Two sexually dimorphic cell groups in the human brain. *Journal of Neuroscience, 9,* 497–506.

Allen, L.., Richey, M. F., Chai, Y. M., Gorski, R. A. (1991). Sex differences in the corpus callosum of the living human being. *Journal of Neuroscience, 11*(4), 933–942.

Amir, S., Waddington, E., Robinson, B., & Stewart, J. (2004). A circadian rhythm in the expression of PERIOD2 protein reveals a novel SCN-controlled oscillator in the oval nucleus of the bed nucleus of the stria terminalis. *Journal of Neuroscience, 24,* 781–790.

Bancila, M., Giuliano, F., Rampin, O., Mailly, P., Brisorguell, M., & Verge, D. (2002). *European Journal of Neuroscience, 16,* 1240–1248.

Bell, E., Willson, M., Wilman, A., Dave, S., & Silverstone, P. (2006). Males and females differ in brain activation during cognitive tasks. *Neuroimage, 30,* 529–538.

Berglund, H., Lindstrom, P., Dhejne-Helmy, C., & Savic, I. (2008). Male-to-female transsexuals show sex-atypical hypothalamus activation when smelling odorous steroids. *Cerebral Cortex, 18,* 1900–1908.

Byne, W., Tobet, S., Mattiace, L. A., Lasco, M. S., Kemether, E., Edgar, M. A., . . . Jones, L. B. (2001). The interstitial nuclei of the human anterior hypothalamus: An investigation of variation with sex, sexual orientation and HIV status. *Hormones and Behavior, 40,* 86–92.

Chung, W., De Vries, G., & Swaab, D. (2002). Sexual differentiation of the bed nucleus of the stria terminalis in humans may extend into adulthood. *Journal of Neuroscience, 22,* 1027–1033.

Clarke, J., & Zaidel, E. (1994). Anatomical-behavioral relationships: Corpus callosum morphometry and hemispheric specialization. *Behavioral Brain Research, 54,* 185–202.

De Lacoste-Utamsing, C., & Holloway, R. (1982). Sexual dimorphism in the human corpus callosum. *Science, 216,* 1431–1432.

Emory, L., Williams, D., Cole, C., Amparo, E., & Meyer, W. (1991). Anatomic variation of the corpus callosum in persons with gender dysphoria. *Archives of Sexual* Behavior, *20,* 409–411.

Garcia-Falgueras, A., & Swaab, D. (2008). A sex difference in the hypothalamic uncinate nucleus: Relationship to gender identity. *Brain, 131,* 3132–3146.

Gelez, H., Poirer, S., Facchinetti, P., Allers, K., Wayman, C., Alexandre, L., & Giulianò, F. (2010). Neuroanatomical evidence for a role of central melanocortin-4 receptors and oxytocin in the efferent control of the rodent clitoris and vagina. *Journal of Sexual Medicine, 7*, 2056–2067.

Gizewski, E., Krause, E., Schlamann, M., Happich, F., Ladd, M. E., Forsting, M., & Senf, W. (2009). Specific cerebral activation due to visual erotic stimuli in male-to-female transsexuals compared with male and female controls: An fMRI study. *Journal of Sexual Medicine, 6*, 440–448.

Gizewski, E., Krause, E., Wanke, I., Forsting, M., & Senf, W. (2006). Gender-specific cerebral activation during cognitive tasks using functional MRI: Comparison of women in mid-luteal phase and men. *Neuroradiology, 48*, 14–20.

Guillamón, A., Segovia, S. & del Abril, A. (1998). Early effects of gonadal steroids on the neuron number in the medial posterior region and the lateral division of the bed nucleus of the stria terminalis in the rat. *Developmental Brain Research, 44*, 281–290.

Kruijver, F. P. M., Zhou, J. N., Pool, C. W., Hofman, M. A., Gooren, J. G., & Swaab, D. F. (2000). Male-to-female transsexuals have female neuron numbers in a limbic nucleus. *Journal of Clinical Endocrine and Metabolism, 85*, 68–70.

Ku, H., Lin, C. S., Chao, H. T., Tu, P. C., Li, C. T., Cheng, C. M., . . . Hsieh, J. C. (2013). Brain signature characterizing the body-brain-mind axis of transsexuals. *PLoS One, 8*, e70808.

LeVay, S. (1991, August). A difference in hypothalamic structure between heterosexual and homosexual men. *Science, 253*, 1034–1037.

Luders, E., Sánchez, F. J., Gaser, C., Toga, A. W., Narr, K. L., Hamilton, L. S., & Vilain, E. (2009). Regional gray matter variation in male-to-female transsexualism. *Neuroimage, 46*, 904–907.

Merchant, H., Zainos, A., Hernandez, A., Salinas, E., & Romo, R. (1997). Functional properties of primate putamen neurons during the categorization of tactile stimuli. *Journal of Neurophysiology, 77*, 1132–1154.

Pol, H. E. H., Cohen-Kettenis, P. T., Van Haren, N. E. M., Peper, J. S., Brans, R. G. H., Cahn, W., . . . Kahn, R. S. (2006). Changing your sex changes your brain: Influences of testosterone and estrogen on adult human brain structure. *European Journal of Endocrinology, 155*, S107–S114.

Preuss, U. W., Meisenzahl, E. M., Frodl, T., Zetzsche, T., Holder, J., Leinsinger, G., . . . Möller, H. J. (2002). Handedness and corpus callosum morphology. *Psychiatric Research, 115*, 33–42.

Rametti, G., Carillo, B., Gomez-Gil, E., Junque, C., Zubiarre-Elorza, L., Segovia, S., . . . Guillamón, A. (2011a). White matter microstructure in female to male transsexuals before cross-sex hormonal treatment. *Journal of Psychiatric Research, 45*, 199–204.

Rametti, G., Carillo, B., Gómez-Gil, E., Junque, C., Zubiarre-Elorza, L., Segovia, S., . . . Guillamón, A. (2011b). The microstructure of white matter in male to female transsexuals before cross-sex hormonal treatment. A DTI study. *Journal of Psychiatric Research, 45,* 949–954.

Rametti, G., Carillo, B., Gomez-Gil, E., Junque, C., Zubiaurre-Elorza, L., Segovia, S., et al. (2012). Effects of androgenization on the white matter microstructure of female-to-male transsexuals. *Psychoneuroendocrinology, 37,* 1261–1269.

Savic, I., Berglund, H., & Lindstrom, P. (2005). Brain response to putative pheromones in homosexual men. *PNAS, 102,* 7356–7361.

Schöning, S., Engelien, A., Bauer, C., Kugel, H., Kersting, A., Roestel, C., . . . Konrad, C. (2010). Neuroimaging differences in spatial cognition between men and male-to-female transsexuals before and during hormone therapy. *Journal of Sexual Medicine, 7,* 1858–1867.

Steinmetz, H., Janacek, L., Kleinschmidt, A., Schlagen, G., Volkmann, J., & Huang, Y. (1992). Sex but no hand difference in the isthmus of the corpus callosum. *Neurology, 42,* 749–752.

Witelson, S. (1985, August 16). The brain connection: The corpus callosum is larger in left-handers. *Science, 229,* 665–668.

Yakota, Y., Kawamura, Y., & Kameya, Y. (2005). Callosal shapes at the mid-sagittal plane: MRI differences of normal males, normal females, and GID. *Proceedings of IEEE Engineering in Medicine and Biology 27th Annual Conference, 1,* 3055–3058.

Zhou, J., Hofman, M., Gooren, L., & Swaab, D. (1995, November). A sex difference in the human brain and its relation to transsexuality. *Nature, 378,* 68–70.

Zhou, J., Hofman, M., & Swaab, D. (1995). VIP neurons in the human SCN in relation to sex, age, and Alzheimer's disease. *Neurobiology of Aging, 16,* 571–576.

11

Conscious Choice and Spirituality

11.0 INTRODUCTION

What triggers transsexuals and transgender people to come out or to greatly increase their transsexualism and transgenderism (TSTG) behavior despite cultural rejection? Is TSTG a conscious lifestyle choice or a biological imperative? How can science explain two-spirit people who experience multiple gender spirituality? These questions are addressed in this chapter from a scientific point of view.

When life crises occur, transsexuals and transgender people are known to come out or increase their TSTG behavior within their congruent gender behavior category. Examples of such crises include the death of a loved one, a family medical crisis, or the end of a war. Psychiatrists have known for some time that they can induce behavior changes in their patients by putting them into a life crisis. The crises are triggered by reminders of mortality, meaninglessness in life, isolation, and freedom of action. These are called **existential crises**. Existential crises result in increased frequency of TSTG and increased desire for body change to conform to the sex associated with a congruent gender behavior category.

Scientific studies indicate that humans make choices long before they are consciously aware of them. This means that the choice to manifest TSTG behavior, like all other human choices, is not made consciously. Decisions are actually made by subconscious processes, not conscious processes. Subconscious gender behavior predispositions insistently try to affect behavior and can only be postponed by salient aspects of family and important activities. Trying to postpone or attempt to eliminate this insistent predisposition forms the basis for military or marriage flight, as described in Section 9.7, to pursue activities that may result in temporary delay of the expression of TSTG behavior.

Two-spirit transsexuals and transgender people report that they have both masculine and feminine spiritual experiences. Childhood reports of gendered spiritual experiences contributed to the assignment of gender behavior category in Native American cultures where gender systems might have included three or four such categories. Other cultures such as the current Bugis people of Indonesia strictly assign one of five gender behavior categories to people who are intensely spiritual, nonsexual, and serve the spiritual needs of the subculture. This fifth gender is considered to be without sex or gender (see Section 4.4). What can science tell us about such gendered and nongendered spiritual experiences?

11.1 EXISTENTIAL CRISES AND TSTG

As already noted, existential crises are known to trigger increases in frequency of TSTG behavior. Whether it is the death of a spouse, a health crisis, loss of a job, or the end of a war, TSTG behavior is increased and sometimes publicly revealed by such crises. Existential crises refer to states of mind that require immediate resolution. The concept comes from Viktor Frankl, a famous psychiatrist who used to deliberately put his patients in such crises to change their behavior for their own benefit. He would do this by steering the discussion of specific situations, particular to each patient, which would provoke such crises. For example, he would lead a patient into a discussion about death by asking the patient to recall a relative who was now deceased or move patients to think about the meaninglessness of their lives by discussing a meaningless job. Yalom, Brown, and Bloch (1975) cataloged some of these methods. Knowledge of the existential crises effects is also important for health care and mental health professionals who help their patients deal with such crises (Laube, 1977; Murray, 1974).

Yalom (1980) identified four types of existential crises:

- Realization that you will die.
- Realization that life has no intrinsic meaning.
- Realization that we are forever isolated from one another.
- Realization of freedom of action.

Existential crises have effects on transsexual and transgender people who are closeted and keep their TSTG behavior or status a secret. For transgender people, the crisis may provoke a TSTG to stop dressing alone in secret and to go out to a support group. It may also increase the frequency of going to TSTG-friendly clubs and organizational events. Existential crises may trigger complete coming out by transgender people and the desire to begin transsexual transition. Those who are already out may also be affected by increasing the frequency of their TSTG behavior. Finally, existential crises can trigger transsexual transition progression including surgeries to change appearance and TS GPS.

Realization that you are mortal and will someday die can be triggered by the death of a loved one or a close friend. Even the remembrance of loss of life can sometimes trigger a crisis. Many TSTG increase their frequency of TSTG behavior after the death of a spouse because they realize that they, too, are mortal and have a limited time to live. A secondary outcome of such deaths is that their deceased spouse or loved one will not be embarrassed by a change in TSTG behavior, which tends to facilitate increases in TSTG behavior. Older transsexuals and transgender people who may have been delaying a change in their TSTG behavior may also come to the realization that they do not have much time to experience their lives authentically.

Realization that life has no intrinsic meaning, only the meaning you give it, can trigger an increase in the frequency of TSTG behavior. Events such as the end of a war, leaving the military, concluding a long-term project, or retirement can provoke an existential crisis. Such events force older transsexuals and transgender people and others to realize that the activities that gave their lives meaning are now gone. A secondary outcome of retirement is that transsexuals and transgender people can also avoid many forms of discrimination that may facilitate a change—for example, if the TSTG has adequate retirement benefits. Chapter 9 included discussions of the tendency of TSTG to engage in high-risk occupations, such as the military or firefighting, and to get married, both of which are both culturally acceptable but require concentration to succeed. Concentration provides a welcome distraction from the insistence of subconscious gender predisposition. An existential crisis forces transsexuals and transgender people to find new activities to give their life purpose and meaning, such as TSTG advocacy or charity.

Realization that we are all isolated from one another is the third existential crisis. We enter and leave this world alone and yet seek to become part of a whole. Divorce and separation may trigger this type of crisis, as may death. Many people cope with isolation crisis by military or marriage flight, which provides companionship and comradeship (see Section 9.7). Isolation crises may cause transsexual or transgender individuals to seek out like-minded people to obtain information and understand who they are. They may now reach out to one another through Internet social media, conferences, and support groups.

Realization of freedom of action means that individuals realize they are responsible for the whole world and its problems and have the freedom of action to improve it. A person is the only author or architect of their own world. If there is something about the world that is wrong, then an individual has a responsibility to fix it because he or she is free to do so. As an existential crisis, realization of freedom of action has been likened to being at the edge of an abyss. Many who became TSTG advocates and support group leaders have probably experienced this existential crisis in combination with the crisis of meaninglessness.

Transsexual and transgender people have increasingly exercised their freedom of action to appear publicly, including media appearances, and to campaign for their civil rights. Transsexual and transgender people now openly lobby at the federal, state, and local level and use lawsuits when necessary to obtain their rights. Because TSTG occurs across all socioeconomic and labor categories, it turns out that many TSTG have particular skills in law, medicine, technology, science, and activism that can aid advocacy. Transsexual and transgender people may not always be visible, but they are ubiquitous. Many feel that they must increase their visibility to be understood, just as many gay and lesbians have come out. Some transsexuals have come out of stealth mode and emerged in the TSTG community to help improve visibility.

It is common for people to experience more than one type of existential crisis at a time from a single or multiple life events. This also applies to transsexual and transgender people. For example, the death of a spouse may create the realization of death, feelings of isolation, and loss of life meaning. Employment discrimination signals isolation from previous coworkers and loss of meaning in life for those dedicated to their jobs. For some transsexuals, genital plastic surgery signals the end of their connections to the TSTG community as they go into stealth mode; transsexual and transgender friends grieve their loss. Because we are required to shape the world by our freedom of action, death means that we have limited time to accomplish our goals.

Many people change their behavior in reaction to existential crises, including transsexuals and transgender people who may greatly increase their frequency of TSTG behavior, engage in voluntary body masculinization/feminization change, increase their visibility, or increase TSTG rights advocacy. To help deal with existential crises, especially isolation, transsexual and transgender people have built communication networks using available media, starting at the mid-20th century (see Section 4.3).

11.2 LIFESTYLE CHOICE VERSUS BIOLOGICAL IMPERATIVE

Some who oppose TSTG civil rights often say that TSTG is just a conscious lifestyle choice and not a biological imperative. They maintain that transsexual and transgender people could easily decide to no longer pursue TSTG behavior and that they could be "cured" by sheer willpower. This section provides some of the scientific evidence that human beings do not have such conscious choice, so the "lifestyle" characterization and "willpower" evocation are untenable positions. This book has presented evidence that TSTG is a biological phenomenon that involves an innate gender behavior predisposition. Such predispositions, like all human predispositions, are expressed through subconscious functions in the brain. The feelings of incongruency for one's assigned gender behavior category can be postponed, but they never go away. As we shall see in this section, subconscious representation of gender behavior predisposition always gets a vote.

11.2.1 Mechanisms in the Nervous System

Most of our nervous system consists of various mechanisms or widgets that we inherited from our biological forebears and are subconscious in nature. Because these widgets were evolutionarily useful or at least did not interfere with reproduction, many of them were passed down to us. For example, we have a biological clock in a small nucleus at the base of the brain, suprachiasmatic nucleus (SCN), which provides the time to set diurnal rhythms in the rest of the brain. We discussed this widget in connection with the discussion of the bed nucleus of the stria terminalis (BNST) in Section 10.1.1 because the resonation of this widget is passed directly to the BNST (Amir, Waddington, Robinson, & Stewart, 2004). The cell group includes an oscillating mechanism that functions like the quartz crystal in some clocks to keep time like an hourglass. We can sense diurnal rhythms from being tired and, to some extent, control them by altering our schedules and exposure to light. The SCN receives inputs directly from the retina of the eye. However, we cannot control our diurnal rhythm by consciously thinking about it.

We have a mechanism in the lower brain stem that mediates motion sickness based on sensory inputs from the eyes and the motion-sensing apparatus in the ear. We cannot control this widget, although when we become sick, we become conscious of nausea and vertigo. There is a nearby nucleus that triggers nausea. Sometimes we really wish that we could control these mechanisms by consciously thinking about them, but we cannot.

Further down in the brain are the widgets that control breathing and other functions. These are the mechanisms that regulate our internal environment. We have limited conscious control of them, although in some cases, such as breathing, there are dual controls—one from the brain stem and one from our consciousness functions. The brain stem mechanism takes over when we do not exert conscious control of breathing while we are conscious of something else or when we are unconscious.

The continuous visual world we see is an illusion. While we perceive the visual world as continuous, visual information acquired by our eyes is highly discontinuous and distorted. There are subconscious widgets in the brain stem that control our eye movements that occur as frequently as 50 per second. The eyes momentarily stop, fixate, and then move on, like they are taking snapshots. The images also are not very sharp when they hit the retina because the cells that sense light face backward at the back of the retina and are obstructed by various nerve and other cells from the light. The visual system in the back of the brain is capable of sharpening each snapshot. There are additional widgets in the visual system that sharpen each snapshot and integrate these discontinuous "snapshots" into an illusion of a continuous visual world.

It turns out that the subconscious widgets in the lower brain can actually guide behavior, even though the visual cortex is damaged and the patient cannot consciously see. This phenomenon is known as **blind sight**. These lower structures, but not the visual cortex, are present in birds and other species and they manage to function quite well with respect to vision. Indeed, many birds have better vision in some respects than humans.

Why does our body deal in illusions? Imagine our panic if we suddenly had to perceive and consciously control the working of all the visual mechanisms in the nervous system and be consciously responsible to process the images to make them into a continuous picture. The world would seem to jump around, and we would have to consciously concentrate to hold it still. We could do nothing else, and it would be overwhelming and inefficient. It would require a much larger brain just to contain the visual system and its conscious connections, which would limit capacity for other functions.

We experience many other illusions including memory recall and motor skills, all of which use unconscious mechanisms, although we sometimes have later conscious experience of them. Like the illusions described here, conscious choice is also an illusion.

11.2.2 The Illusion of Conscious Choice

Like the illusion of continuous visual space, conscious choice is another illusion created by our nervous system (Jaynes, 2000). We know this from the results of some of the first psychological experiments, and we now know it from cognitive neuroscience research, using neurophysiological measurements.

Consciousness is the awareness of events and decisions. It sometimes is described as an "inner voice" or "stream of consciousness" that narrates experience. Used in this sense, it is different from being conscious or from being unconscious due to injury or sleep.

One of the oldest yet simplest psychological experiments was conducted in Wurzburg, Germany, in the late 19th century by some of the first psychologists. Anyone can conduct this experiment for themselves. Just take two objects—say, a pen and a pencil—and hold one in each hand. Now judge which is heavier. You will find that the decision as to which is heavier is made subconsciously. You can later be consciously aware of the sensation of each object on your hand, but the decision is already made for you. Just as with the illusion of continuous vision, if you were aware of all the subconscious mechanisms that contribute to this simple choice, you would be overwhelmed. Our illusions of choice protect us from that panic. We are now beginning to learn from cognitive neuroscience how these illusions are performed.

Cognitive neuroscience experiments confirm that the awareness of choice occurs well after the choice is made by our subconscious mechanisms, just as with the Wurzburg choice experiment. Conscious choice is an illusion—we have already made the decision prior to us becoming conscious of it. We are just now beginning to understand these mechanisms through measurements of brain activity and real-time brain scanning technology.

While recording electroencephalogram (EEG) during decision tasks, Libet, Gleason, Wright, and Pearl (1983) found a cerebral electrical signal that preceded conscious awareness of decision making by at least half a second. The EEG measures electrical potentials from many active neurons, mostly in the cerebral cortex. The decisions tested in the Libet experiment were self-initiated decisions to move while the EEG was being recorded. Libet, Ghewon, Wright, and Pearl (1983) concluded that subconscious processes that preceded conscious awareness in time actually made the decision. Keller and Heckhausen (1990) found that similar potentials occurred before an unconscious movement as well. Libet (1993) later found that decisions made conscious included a delay, indicating that consciousness awareness actually delayed the act. This is presumably because being conscious of a decision activated subconscious mechanisms that caused the delay. Trevena and Miller (2002) found that although the subconscious decision for motor movement was made before it became conscious, the actual motor preparation to move sometimes occurred after the decision became conscious. Subconscious mechanisms were implementing the decision. Finally, Guggisberg and Mottaz (2013) found that there were indications that consciousness decision took a gradual buildup to complete.

With the advent of fMRI technology, activation of parts of the brain can be identified and measured in real time. Functional magnetic resonance imaging (fMRI) measures either increases in blood flow in regions of the brain or water flow in the fiber bundles of neurons of brain, depending on the type of scan. The use of fMRI extends our ability to identify parts of the brain that are involved in decision making. The frontal and parietal (side) cortices appear to be the main structures involved. Lesion studies indicate involvement by the frontal lobes (Bechara & Van Der Linden, 2005; Fellows, 2006; Fellows, 2011). Numerous fMRI and other studies indicate that the frontal lobes are involved in value decisions (Gluth, Rieskamp, & Buchel, 2012; Volz, Schubotz, & von

Cramon, 2006; Zysset, Huber, Ferstl, & von Cramon, 2002), ethical decisions (Heekeren, Wartenburger, Schmidt, Schwintowski, & Villringer, 2003), and complex free decisions (Soon, Brass, Heinze, & Haynes, 2008), and task switching (Bode et al., 2009).

Soon, Brass, Heinz, & Haynes (2008) found that decisions had already been made subconsciously in the prefrontal and parietal cortices at least 10 seconds before conscious awareness for free decisions. Bode et al. (2011) found that a decision could be decoded in the lateral prefrontal cortex and parietal lobe before it reached awareness. Soon, Brass, Heinz, & Haynes (2008) also found that the outcome of a decision could be predicted at least 4 seconds before conscious awareness for more abstract decisions (mathematical decisions) in the medial prefrontal cortex and the parietal cortex. Supporting these results are reports from recording single neuronal units in the human medial prefrontal area, which indicate that recruitment of cells starts at least 1,500 msec (1,500 thousandths of a second) before a decision and that there is sufficient activity evidence that will predict a movement 700 msec before conscious awareness.

There are examples from infrahuman species that indicate that a "population coding" or "vector voting scheme" may be at work in the cortex during the subconscious decision process. Neurons "fire" when they transmit information to the next neuron by a chemical disturbance that moves through the external surface of the neuron. Firing involves a large change in the surface chemistry. In population or vector voting functional organizations, each neuron is coded to fire representing a different alternative and can also vary its frequency of firing rate. The higher the frequency, the more influence that individual neuron has on the decision. In a series of elegant experiments, Georgopoulos et al. (Georgopoulos, 1991; Georgopoulos, Lunito, Petrides, Schwartz, & Massey, 1989; Georgopoulos, Schwartz, & Kettner, 1986) found that a population coding scheme predicted the behavior of rhesus monkeys to move a joystick in a designated direction to obtain a reward. The recordings were in the premotor area of the cortex, but this "population coding" or "vector voting" scheme appears to be a common neural approach to coordination of subconscious mechanisms including decision making.

As applied to TSTG, the evidence on decision making in the brain indicates that subconscious mechanisms "vote" on behavior. Among these subconscious mechanisms may be one that expresses gender predisposition and is constantly comparing gender predisposition with the behaviors of a person's assigned gender behavior category. Subconscious gender predisposition gets a vote on behavior. Other subconscious mechanisms may compete in the voting, but the gender behavior predisposition does not go away. We may not understand what bothers us about an incongruent assigned gender behavior category, but it will always have a vote in the subconscious decision-making process. Mechanisms representing other potential behaviors may compete with it, but gender predisposition processes never go away.

11.3 ETHEREAL SPIRITS AND SPIRITUAL EXPERIENCE

The two-spirit tradition of the Native Americans for multiple gender behavior categories indicates that transsexuals and transgender people have both masculine and feminine spirits that inspire TSTG behavior (see Section 4.2). Therefore, an ethereal spirit might be gendered. This is similar to the problem of whether there is an ethereal soul or a body-disconnected "mind" that guides human behavior. These issues have been debated and researched for centuries.

There is no scientific evidence that there are ethereal spirits that communicate with us through our brains to create behavior. Logically, this requires an interface between ethereal spirits and the physical brain. Descartes (1664/2003) suggested that the "seat of the soul" was in the **pineal body** because it was one of the few structures that straddles both brain hemispheres and therefore might be able to control both. In his view, the pineal body was supposed to be the seat of the soul and the interface between the ethereal spirits and the nervous system. Since Descartes, scientists have mapped the brain and explored its functionality for many centuries, but no interface has been found that can communicate with an ethereal spirit or a soul, including the pineal body. The pineal body appears to be involved in diurnal rhythms.

The postulation of ethereal spirits that work through the brain to guide behavior is self-contradictory. The interface between the ethereal spirit and the corporeal body cannot be either ethereal or corporeal. If the interface were ethereal, then it would have to be partly corporeal to communicate with the brain, but this violates the principle that it is ethereal and having no substance. If it is corporeal, then it cannot communicate with an ethereal spirit without being partially ethereal, which is contradictory to things corporeal. Such an interface would either violate the nonphysicality of the spirit or violate the laws of physical matter.

Because science is constantly discovering new things, we cannot absolutely rule out the existence of an interface between ethereal spirits and the body, but we have not found such an interface to date. At this point, we must assume that the perception of spiritual experience is mediated by subconscious mechanism(s) in the nervous system rather than through extracorporeal spirits. As we saw in the last section, many subconscious mechanisms get to vote on behavior.

We need not question the value or reports of spiritual experience, but we need not assume that spirituality is mediated by nonphysical mechanisms. Spiritual experience appears to be one of the uniquely human functions that provide comfort and inspiration. We should respect spirituality but also seek to understand it scientifically.

Spiritual experience refers to the inspiration that one receives from internal experiences, but it does not necessarily involve ethereal spirits, souls, or religion. Experiences such as seeing the Milky Way on a clear night inspire us by evoking the awe at the vastness of the cosmos and its interdependencies. Spiritual experience can come from within through meditation or just being mindful about existential issues. At this point in science, we might assume that the "two-spirits" experience comes from subconscious brain mechanisms that may represent two different gender predispositions. These mechanisms may give us an experience of dual spirituality, but the source of these experiences is not ethereal spirits but rather subconscious mechanisms.

11.4 SUMMARY

Transsexuals and transgender people may come out or greatly increase their TSTG behavior because they experience existential crises. All people may change their behavior because of existential crises. It appears that TSTG is a biological imperative that works on a subconscious level to influence behavior. As far as can currently be known through science, gendered spirituality comes from more than one subconscious brain mechanism, rather than from more than one ethereal spirit. Nevertheless, spirituality is of great importance and should continue to be studied scientifically because it is a valuable and common human experience.

REFERENCES

Amir, S., Waddington, E., Robinson, B., & Stewart, J. (2004). A circadian rhythm in the expression of PERIOD2 protein reveals a novel SCN-controlled oscillator in the oval nucleus of the bed nucleus of the stria terminalis. *Journal of Neuroscience, 24,* 781–790.

Bechara, A., & Van Der Linden, M. (2005). Decision-making and impulse control after frontal lobe injuries. *Current Opinion in Neurology, 18,* 734–739.

Bode, S., He, A. H., Soon, C. S., Trampel, R., Turner, R., & Haynes, J.-D. (2011). Tracking the unconscious generation of free decisions using ultra-high field fMRI. *PLoS One, 6,* e21612.

Descartes, R. (2003). *Treatise on man.* Amherst, NY: Prometheus. (Original work published 1664.)

Fellows, K. (2006). Deciding how to decide: Ventromedial frontal lobe damage affects information acquisition in multi-attribute decision-making. *Brain, 124,* 944–952.

Fellows, L. (2011). Orbitofrontal contributions to value-base decision making: Evidence from humans with frontal lobe damage. *Annals of the New York Academy of Science, 1239,* 51–58.

Georgopoulos, A. (1991). Higher order motor control. *Annual Reviews in Neuroscience, 14,* 361–377.

Georgopoulos, A., Lunito, J., Petrides, M., Schwartz, A., & Massey, J. (1989). Mental rotation of the neuronal population vector. *Science, 243,* 234–236.

Georgopoulos, A., Schwartz, A., & Kettner, R. (1986). Neuronal population coding of movement directions. *Science, 233,* 1416–1419.

Gluth, S., Rieskamp, J., & Buchel, C. (2012). Deciding when to decide: Time-variant sequential models explain the emergence of value-based decisions in the human brain. *Journal of Neuroscience, 32,* 10686–10698.

Guggisberg, A., & Mottaz, A. (2013). Timing and awareness of movement decisions: Does consciousness really come too late? *Frontiers of Human Neuroscience, 3,* 385.

Heekeren, H., Wartenburger, I., Schmidt, H., Schwintowski, H., & Villringer, A. (2003). An fMRI study of simple ethical decision-making. *Neuroreport, 14,* 1215–1219.

Jaynes, J. (2000). *The origin of consciousness in the breakdown of the bicameral mind.* New York: Houghton Mifflin Harcourt.

Keller, I., & Heckhausen, H. (1990). Readiness potentials proceeding spontaneous motor acts: Voluntary v. involuntary control. *Electroencephalography and Clinical Neurophysiology, 76,* 351–361.

Laube, J. (1977). Death and dying workshop for nurses. *International Journal of Nursing Students, 14,* 111–120.

Libet, B. (1993). The neural factor in conscious and unconscious events. *Ciba Foundation Symposium, 174,* 123–137.

Libet, B., Gleason, C., Wright, E., & Pearl, D. (1983). Time of conscious intention to act in relation to onset of cerebral activity (readiness-potential). The unconscious initiation of a freely voluntary act. *Brain, 106,* 623–642.

Murray, P. (1974). Death education and its effect on the death anxiety level of nurses. *Psychological Reports, 35,* 1250.

Soon, C., Brass, M., Heinze, H., & Haynes, J. (2008). Unconscious determinant of free decisions in the human brain. *Nature Neuroscience, 11,* 543–545.

Trevena, J., & Miller, J. (2002). Cortical movement preparation before and after a conscious decision to move. *Conscious Cognition, 11,* 162–190.

Volz, K., Schubotz, R., & von Cramon, D. (2006). Decision-making and the frontal lobes. *Current Opinion in Neurology, 19,* 401–406.

Yalom, I. (1980). *Existential psychotherapy.* New York: Basic Books.

Yalom, I., Brown, S., & Bloch, S. (1975). The written summary as a group psychotherapy technique. *Archives of General Psychiatry, 302,* 605–613.

Zysset, S., Huber, O., Ferstl, E., & von Cramon, D. (2002). The anterior fronto-median cortex and evaluative judgment: An fMRI study. *Neuroimage, 15,* 983–991.

Psychopathology

12.0 INTRODUCTION

This chapter provides a historical discussion of past psychopathological causation theories of transsexualism and transgenderism (TSTG). Today, scientific evidence is being used to develop nonpathological theories of TSTG, which can help to understand the phenomenon and reduce the rejection of transsexuals and transgender people. The future will bring even greater technological capabilities to measure brain mechanisms involved in TSTG.

Mental health providers were the first professionals to deal with the problems affecting transsexuals and transgender people. In their schooling, these providers were trained to apply the "medical model," which requires identification of an underlying pathology before an appropriate treatment can be selected. For this reason, they hypothesized psychopathological theories of TSTG to rationalize treatments. The problem with most such theories is that they do not qualify as scientific theories. They cannot be "**operationalized**" or defined in sufficient objective detail to generate specific testable hypotheses. They rely on intervening variables that cannot be measured. Some predict all possible outcomes. Some invent post hoc historical psychological events to retroactively explain outcomes and behavior. They therefore are not scientific or evidence-based.

All this is not to castigate mental health professionals for doing the best that they could. They did not yet have the tools to measure events in the brain and nervous system. Now all that is changing. We have instrumentation to scan the brain and watch it function in real time. The brain is actually a chemical computer, and we also now have more precise pharmacological agents to explore its chemistry. We can make direct electrical measurements of neural activity in small areas of the brain in unanesthetized people. And we have immense computer power to analyze all these measurements.

We have just scratched the surface of applying these research technologies to TSTG because of cultural rejection of the phenomena and because research money is often allocated to particular diseases. Since TSTG violates cultural norms but is not a disease, budgets to study TSTG are meager. For this reason, pathological theories of TSTG have not disappeared. The discussion of such theories in the public forum continues to pathologize transsexuals and transgender people, which reinforces cultural rejection. The pathologization of TSTG continues to interfere with understanding it because it prevents funding for research. If mental health professionals continue to discuss TSTG as if it were pathological, they are encouraging themselves to think about TSTG as a disorder or disease. Likewise, if mental health professionals and others continue to discuss TSTG in the public forum as if it were pathological, public understanding will continue to be blocked.

In recent years, there has been a movement to depathologize TSTG. One objective of this effort has been to change the compilations of mental health insurance reimbursement codes, including the *Diagnostic and Statistical Manual of Mental Disorders* (DSM), which is compiled by the American Psychiatric Association. In 2013, an effort was made to depathologize TSTG in the 5th edition of the DSM, but the effort was not as successful as it was said to be in the press.

A portion of the World Health Organization's **International Classification of Diseases** (ICD) is the equivalent of the DSM outside the United States, and its main objective is to standardize terminology worldwide for reporting and monitoring and to improve research communication. On October 1, 2015, the 10th edition of the ICD (ICD-10) will supersed the DSM-V in the United States to comply with health care privacy legislation. The relevant portion of the current version of ICD is similar to DSM-IV with regard to TSTG diagnoses. It is currently under revision, and the outcome for TSTG in the upcoming ICD-11 has yet to be determined. Thus, as of October 2015, the ICD-10 will continue to make TSTG pathological, sidelining changes made to DSM-V; it is unknown how this will change with ICD-11.

Just as mental health professionals who were homosexual and others in the gay, lesbian, and bisexual (GLB) community put intellectual pressure on the mental health community to depathologize homosexuality, the TSTG community has risen up to do the same. However, homosexuality was dropped as a disorder in 1972, whereas TSTG was only temporarily reclassified in 2013.

12.1 PSYCHOPATHOLOGICAL CHARACTERIZATIONS OF TSTG

Although there are probably as many psychopathological characterizations of TSTG as there are mental health professionals who have encountered transsexual or transgender people, this section provides an overview of some of the most common themes. For convenience, 22 psychopathological characterizations of TSTG are grouped into five categories:

- Sexual fetishism
- Parental interactions
- Personality disorder
- Anxiety
- Defense

Each of the psychodynamic characterizations are discussed within these categories in subsequent sections.

12.1.1 Sexual Fetishism

The term **fetish** pertains to sexual arousal from the stimuli of inanimate objects not associated with sexual intercourse. Arousal is not sufficient to make the fetish a disorder because most people get sexually aroused to some extent by such stimuli. For a fetish to be a disorder, it must cause impairment or distress, and it must interfere with social and other functioning. The psychopathological term for fetish is **paraphilia**. The theory of **autogynephilia** is categorized as a fetish or paraphilia theory because of how it has been operationalized for experimentation as described below.

12.1.1.1 Autogynephilia

Autogynephilia is a term coined by Blanchard (1989, 2005) and used by others (Ekins & King, 2001; Lawrence, 2007) to describe an underlying psychodynamic causal factor in MTF TSTG involving "love of oneself as a woman." It is considered by its proponents as a "paraphilia" or fetish, which is a pathological term usually used to describe a mental disorder that involves life disruption and distress. Autogynephilia is highly controversial among transsexuals, transgender people, and mental health professionals because it pathologizes those people who engage in TSTG behavior and because it not a scientific theory. There is scientific evidence that sexual arousal does not seem to be the motivating factor for TSTG. For Blanchard and Lawrence, autogynephilia pertains only to male-to-female (MTF) transsexuals and transgender people who are heterosexual.

The definition of autogynephilia has varied widely:

- "aroused by the thought or image of themselves as a female" (Blanchard (1989).
- "Autogynephilia . . . may find expression in the fantasy of having intercourse, as a woman, with a man" (Blanchard, 1989).
- "[E]rotic arousal in association with the thought or image of themselves as women."
- "Autogynephilia takes a variety of forms. Some men are most aroused sexually by the idea of wearing women's clothes, and they are primarily interested in wearing women's clothes. Some men are most aroused sexually by the idea of having a woman's body, and they are most interested in acquiring a woman's body" (Lawrence, 2006 quoting Blanchard 1989).
- Alternatively as "love of oneself as a woman" (Blanchard, 2005).
- Alternatively as "love of women and want[ing] to become what they love" (Lawrence, 2007).

Blanchard and Lawrence sometimes exclude clothing and feminine behavior from this definition and sometimes substitute romantic arousal for sexual arousal.

Supporters of autogynephilia sometimes maintain that it is not a purely erotic phenomena. They sometimes conceptualize it as a type of sexual orientation and as a variety of romantic love. They believe it involves both erotic and affectional or attachment-based elements (Lawrence, 2007). Most MTF TSTG reject these formulations as inconsistent with their experience.

From the wide variety of definitions, it is clear that the concept of autogynephilia is not well defined and cannot be easily operationalized. For this reason alone, it does not constitute a scientific theory. Scientific evidence exists indicating that love correlates with oxytocin release and nerve growth factor release and that it has neuroanatomical correlates. When the proponents are referring to love, are they referring to oxytocin hormone release or some other biological mechanism of love or pair bonding? When they refer to romance are they referring to Platonic love involving attraction without sexual arousal?

The two attempts to operationalize autogynephilia indicate that the concept really devolves into demonstrations that MTF transsexual and transgender people have learned sexual arousal to feminine clothing and presentation. Their sexual arousal occurs because of their male bodies and their previous experience in learning sexual arousal to objects. Nearly all males and some females have learned such arousal, whether transsexual/transgender or not, as discussed in Chapter 9. The first attempt at operationalization was the development of a scale that purports to measure "core autogynephilia," the other was a TSTG sexual arousal experiment.

As with other psychodynamic theories, the problem with autogynephilia is that it cannot be operationalized sufficiently to conduct experimentation. It therefore does not qualify as a scientific theory or hypothesis. One empirical proof offered by supporters involves a **core autogynephilia scale** (Blanchard, 1989). The instrument asks subjects how they feel about the concept of themselves as a woman. But responses to these questions, as in all concept recall, necessitates recall of attributes (Bruner, Goodnow, & Austin, 1967). This means that if the subject has previously learned sexual arousal responses to attributes of clothing or gender presentation that the concept evokes, then they would become sexually aroused. It is impossible for subjects to respond to some of the questions about the concept of themselves as a woman or the concept of love without visualizing or recalling what a woman looks like or how a woman behaves. For this reason, questionnaire items are not specific enough to exclude how the subject responds to the stimuli of clothing, feminine behavior, or romantic behavior from consideration during subject response.

A physiological phalloplethysmography study is often cited as support for autogynephilia (Blanchard, Racansky, & Steiner, 1986). This study demonstrated that MTF transgender people were sexually aroused by presentation of cross-dressing stories as measured by penile blood pressure. In this study, there was no attempt to actually test autogynephilia or isolate the concepts of the "idea of oneself as a woman" or the "love of oneself as a woman" from the structure of the cross-dressing stories. It is also not surprising that the transgender people responded with sexual arousal to cross-dressing stories. One would expect from classical conditioning extinction theory (see Section 9.3) that the extinction (desensitization) of all of the conditioned stimulus–response connections between feminine clothing and behavior that took many years to establish should take multiple exposures to extinguish. Besides, some arousing stimuli could turn on both males and females, such as cross-dressing or leather or vinyl wear. The Blanchard, Racansky, and Steiner (1986) study provided no empirical support for autogynephilia through its design or results.

In the first peer-reviewed critique of the literature on autogynephilia, Moser (2010) found the following:

- He could not find reports of any substantial difference between the gender dysphoria nonhomosexual (MTF) transsexuals who supposedly had autogynephilia and homosexual transsexuals.
- A substantial percentage (15%–36%) of homosexual transsexuals report sexual arousal to cross-sex dressing and presentation.
- A substantial percentage (10%–27%) of nonhomosexual transsexuals report no sexual arousal to cross-sex dressing and presentation.
- "The purported clinical significance of BAT [autogynephilia] is not clear."

Moser (2010) concluded:

> Contrary to the conclusions of BAT [autogynephilia] proponents, many
> of the tenets of the theory are not supported by the existing data or both
> supporting and contrary data exists. The rejection of the data contrary to
> BAT [autogynephilia] by its proponents raises questions about the valid-
> ity of the other data on which BAT [autogynephilia] is based. (p. 805)

The concept of autogynephilia continues to contribute to the pathologization of transsexual and transgender people. Supporters assert that some types
of MTF TSTG constitute paraphilias, a psychopathological category that has
traditionally included such phenomena as apotemnophilia, voyeurism, zoo-
philia, necrophilia, pedophilia, and kleptophilia. When it is classed with such
bizarre phenomena, transsexuals and transgender people become pathologized. As an example, Lawrence (2006) published an article likening TSTG to
apotemnophilia, which is the desire to amputate a healthy limb. Those in the
public sphere who oppose TSTG rights have used these terms to pathologize
the phenomena.

As would be expected from sexual arousal principles of learning and
extinction (see Section 9.3), there are reports from nonhomosexual TSTG who
comment that they do not get aroused by cross-dressing. These people have
been dismissed by proponents of autogynephilia, saying that these people are
"autogynephiles" who are in denial rather than being open to exploring sexual arousal phenomena. It should also be no surprise that there are reports by
homosexual TSTG who say that they are sexually aroused by cross-dressing.
Learning of sexual arousal depends on experience, and anyone can become
subsequently aroused by most any stimulus.

Reports from TSTG support group surveys indicate that the motivation
for TSTG is not sexual arousal but instead relaxation, comfort, and relief
from the rules of an incongruent gender behavior category (Buhrich, 1978).
Learned sexual arousal can be extinguished or reduced through exposure to
the stimuli but TSTG behavior persists.

12.1.2 Parental Interactions

12.1.2.1 Mother-Child Relations

Only a few years after the introduction of TS genital plastic surgery (GPS)
for transsexuals (then called sexual reassignment surgery) and after publica-
tion of Harry Benjamin's (1966) book on transsexualism, Stoller (1968) published his interpretation of transsexualism. Stoller believed that relationships
between a male and his mother were responsible for transsexualism, although
he believed in a "core gender identity," which was determined by natal biology

and learning similar to imprinting. Both males and females would establish a core gender identity unless the relationship with the mother was disturbed by a masculine influence. He saw MTF transsexualism as occurring through the desires of the mother. Stoller was criticized by Lothstein (1979) for not considering the internal processes of transsexuals to defend themselves.

Lothstein (1979) believed that conflict and defense between parent and child occurs during development and individuation. He suggested that there was a "gender symbiosis" between the mother and MTF male child in which the mother tolerates some separation for masculine behavior but not for gender identity. The attachment to the mother remains through development of a feminine identity for the MTF. With regard to the female to male (FTM), the mother actively pushes her daughters away from the feminine. The transsexual child is able to avoid psychosis and distinguish the self from objects.

Lothstein (1979) cited work by Winnicott (1971) to explain transsexualism. He stated that "The mother–child relationship and the quality of parenting are the bedrock on which gender disturbances rest." Winnicott emphasized development of a "false self" that was internalized as true and that through transitional objects revealed the crossover between reality and fantasy. In applying Winnicott's ideas, Lothstein (1979) maintained that the transsexual develops two selves—a true or secret one internally and a false self externally to avoid conflict with parents and others. The secret, internal self helps the child maintain a separate identity and independence from his or her mother. Transitional objects allow the child to make connections between his or her true self and the phony external false self. For transsexuals, clothing and presentation become transitional objects.

As we saw in Chapter 8, many suspected aspects of the mother-child relationship, including a mother who is too close to the child, are eliminated by empirical evidence, but psychodynamic characterizations of TSTG involving parents are still considered by mental health professionals.

12.1.3 Personality Disorder

Several researchers have characterized TSTG as a personality disorder or as a disorder with frequent co-occurrence of personality disorder.

Using Rorschach testing, Murray (1985) reported that MTF transsexuals met the criteria for borderline personality disorder as defined by Kernberg (1977). Compared with control subjects, transsexuals displayed "more aggression, lower level of object relations, poorer reality testing and impaired boundary differentiation." Transsexuals did not differ significantly from a borderline personality group. Murray concluded that MTF should be included in the borderline personality disorder category. Bodlund (1993) found in the Structured Clinical Interview for DSM-III (SCID) that 5 of 19 transsexuals showed personality disorders and pathology in 8 of 12 personality trait categories. Co-occurrence of TSTG with psychiatric illness was also assessed by Hepp, Kraemer, Schnyder, Miller, and Delsignore (2005) using the SCID interview. The transsexuals showed signs of Axis I disorders, anxiety, mood disorders, and substance-related disorders. Given that transsexuals are anxious and upset from cultural and family rejection, these results are not surprising but also are not pathological. Because none of the transsexuals had previously been diagnosed with Axis I disorders, the authors concluded that transsexual and transgender people belong in their own diagnostic category and that personality disorder was not a precondition for developing TSTG.

Another Rorschach study, this time with adolescent transsexuals (Cohen, Ruiter, Ringelberg, & Cohen-Kettenis, 1997), found that psychopathology was not required for the development of transsexualism. Finally, using a symptom checklist and the DSM-III SCID, Haraldsen and Dahl (2000) found that transsexuals selected for TS GPS showed a low level of psychopathology before and after surgery. The SCID was the same as that used in the Bodlund study. Haraldson and Dahl (2000) concluded: "This finding casts doubt on the view that transsexualism is a severe mental disorder" (p. 276).

Use of the Rorschach test has been questioned, particularly because of its high false-positive error rate in some categories of interpretation (Wood, Lilienfeld, Garb, & Nezworski, 2000; Wood, Nezworski, Lilienfeld, & Garb, 2003) and its validity (Wood et al., 2010); others have noted the difficulties inherent in aggregating data from already low-validity individual results (Garb, Wood, Lilienfeld, & Nezworski, 2005). Taken together, these results indicate that TSTG is not due to an inherent personality disorder.

12.1.3.1 Dissociation

People play many roles in their lives—parent, coach, student, employee, and a variety of social roles. Personality as a mode of responding changes with these roles. It is only when a person cannot remember events that occurred in another role that **dissociation** is involved. Dissociation is believed to be caused by childhood abuse. There have been suggestions that TSTG is a form of dissociation because many transsexuals and transgender people, particularly those who live in partial secrecy, play roles that vary in terms of their adherence to multiple gender behavior categories. What researchers found was that although dissociation was not present in transsexuals, many of the transsexuals had a history of child abuse. Chapter 8 addressed the issue of abuse and noted that TSTG children were abused because of their TSTG behavior. Devor (1994) interviewed 45 FTM transsexuals and found that many showed signs of childhood abuse. She did not conclude that FTM transsexuals are dissociative.

Saks (1998) reported a case study of a single FTM transsexual who had been abused as a child and had both masculine and feminine personalities.

The patient reports loss of memory even at an early age. Using a screening test for dissociation, the Dissociative Experiences Scale (DES), Wailing, Goodwin, and Cole, (1998) found that 10% of the transsexuals tested scored above 30 on this test. This test does not claim high predictive validity, however. Only 17% of people diagnosed as dissociative have scores greater than 30.

Kersting et al. (2003) found that neither the DES nor the SCID could be used to screen or classify transsexuals as being dissociative. The study group included 29 MTF and 12 FTM transsexuals. On the DES scale, transsexuals did score higher than controls, but this was due entirely to a single item on the 28-item scale: "Some people have the experience of feeling that their body—or parts of their body—does not seem to belong to them." The researchers concluded that responses on this question for transsexualism were not a sign of dissociation but might be a sign of transsexualism. Kersting et al. (2003) did find that nearly half (48%) of the transsexuals tested reported childhood emotional abuse.

What is striking about these studies (Devor, 1994; Kersting et al., 2003) are the reports of TSTG child abuse that do not seem to cause dissociation. Although some transsexuals have been diagnosed with dissociation, there is little evidence to believe that TSTG is due to dissociation or child abuse.

12.1.3.2 Warding Off Personality Decompensation

Lothstein (1979) suggested that the reason reparative therapy does not work for transsexuals is due to personality decompensation. Decompensation means that transsexuals do not form the core gender identity required by cultural norms for their sex. Instead, to shield their defective core gender identity, they form an opposite-sex gender identity that is defective. Therapists who try to change the gender identification of transsexuals may find that there is no core to go back to and no gender structures to fall back on (Socarides, 1970).

Because all of the ideas involved in personality decompensation are poorly defined intervening variables, it is impossible to operationalize and empirically test this theory.

12.1.3.3 Stigmatized Homosexuality

Because historically culture stigmatized homosexuality before transsexuality, the idea that TSTG behavior is a result of homosexuality still exists. So the idea goes (Lothstein, 1979), there are some homosexuals who seek transsexual transition because they cannot tolerate the stigma from being homosexual and wanting a pair bond and sexual arousal from a same-sex person. The idea is that transsexuals are perceived to be heterosexual, which is more culturally acceptable. According to the idea, culture views transsexualism more kindly.

Of course, since Lothstein's time, homosexuality has become more acceptable in most parts of the world. We also know that transsexuals may retain their attraction for opposite natal-sex partners even after transition and TS GPS. However, the idea that TSTG is caused by homosexuality lives on with some mental health professionals as well as some of the public. This idea is advanced by those who seek to dismiss transsexuals and transgender people as merely homosexuals.

Homosexuality appears to be an independent phenomenon from TSTG. Homosexuality has been found to run in families, but heritability of homosexuality is low in twin studies. Research including a full genome scan found genetic markers for homosexuality in the Xq28 region and the 7q36, 8p12, and 10q26 regions (Hamer, Hu, Hu, Magnusone, & Pattatuchi 1993; Hu et al., 1995; Kruglyak & Lander, 1995; Mustanski et al., 2005; Turner, 1995), which are different marker locations than either MTF or FTM TSTG (see Section 5.3). Although there is some dispute about whether there is a genetic marker for homosexuality, the results of a full scan rule out an association with TSTG. Attention is now turning to potential epigenetic causal mechanisms for homosexuality (Rice, Friberg, & Gavrilets, 2012), and so far no overlap with TSTG mechanisms has been reported. Homosexuality can co-occur with TSTG. As we saw in Chapter 6 from sibling sex ratios, sibling birth numbers, and sibling birth order studies, there appears to be an epigenetic imprinting mechanism for homosexuality.

12.1.4 Anxiety

The concepts of male castration anxiety and female penis envy were originated by Freud (1950/1977), who suggested that they originated in children during the period from 3 to 5 years of age. Male children were anxious about losing their penis, and females were envious that male children had penises. The concepts were broadened to reflect the relationship of children to interpersonal power.

The application of castration anxiety to TSTG meant that males would preemptively castrate themselves to reduce anxiety. Likewise, females seek a penis to reduce their anxiety about being powerless. Although MTF transsexuals denied castration anxiety, Lothstein (1979) interpreted their Rorschach test responses to indicate body defectiveness and a distorted body image. In this same study, FTM responses in the Rorschach test were interpreted as involving the belief that they already had a penis.

The frequency of male castration is more than 44,000 per year; the main reason is for treating prostate cancer. In an online survey, few transsexual or transgender people mentioned any interest in castration (Wassersug, Zeleniectz, & Squire 2004). There is interest in voluntary castration outside of prostate cancer treatment or TS GPS (Wassersug, Zeleniectz, & Squire 2004), but it is hard to judge the reason why or the seriousness of people from an online survey.

Because all of the ideas involved in castration anxiety and penis envy are poorly defined intervening variables, it is difficult to operationalize and empirically test this theory. The available evidence indicates that transsexuals do not seek transition and TS GPS and that transgender people do not cross-dress because of castration anxiety or penis envy.

12.1.5 Defense

Psychodynamic ideas have been developed that explain TSTG in terms of identity defense by repression, denial, or fantasy.

12.1.5.1 Identity Defense

Veale (2010) emphasized that repression was involved in the delay of transsexuals and transgender people to deal with their "gender-variant" identities. He included motivated forgetting and lack of awareness in repression. Veale cites studies of young children who mainly use denial to defend against anxiety-provoking information. Older children and adults may use repression defenses.

Although transsexuals and transgender people may resist performing TSTG behavior by military or marriage flight or engaging in other activities, there is no indication that biological gender predisposition goes away because of an active forgetting mechanism. Gender predisposition is an unlearned biological mechanism and not one learned through experience or lost through forgetting.

As we observed in Chapter 8, although the realization of TSTG or at least the recognition that something is wrong with gender behavior category assignment may start at age 4, it may take years before TSTG behavior appears or a person realizes that they are transsexual or transgender (Lawrence, 2003). Sometimes this uneasy feeling lasts into adulthood. Once TSTG is realized, the psychology of secrecy (Kelly, 2002) begins to take effect with the person constantly calculating to defend himself or herself, which would make denial and repression impossible to occur.

12.1.5.2 Snow White Syndrome

Some mental health practitioners believe that TSTG can be attributed to the Snow White syndrome. This syndrome refers to a form of defense in which the patient hides in a world of fantasy and make believe to obtain protection from the self-motivated desire for castration (Michel & Mormont, 2002). As transsexual transition progresses, the need for escape into fantasy decreases (Michel & Mormont, 2004). The authors rely on the Rorschach inkblot test evidence for proof of the Snow White syndrome. However, as noted earlier, the Rorschach test has been criticized for its subjectivity and lack of validity (Lilienfeld, Wood, & Garb, 2000; Wood et al., 2010). In particular, as noted earlier, the validity of the Rorschach test has been questioned because of its high false-positive error rate in some categories of interpretation (Wood et al., 2001a; Wood 2001b) and because there are difficulties inherent in aggregating data from already low-validity individual results (Garb, Wood, Liftenfeld, & Nezwarski 2005). After a 5-year study of the Rorschach, Wood et al. (2003) concluded that it was of little value for personality testing or mental diagnosis.

The suggestion of the Snow White syndrome suffers from the same problems as other psychopathological theories in that it posits intervening variables that cannot be measured and cannot be used to make predictions.

12.2 DSM-V AND ICD-11

As discussed earlier, in recent years, there has been a movement to depathologize transsexualism and transgenderism by both TSTG advocates and professional organizations such as WPATH. One of the objectives of this movement is to depathologize the lists of mental disorders compiled by the American Psychiatric Association and international organizations. These categories are used by hate mongers and those opposed to acceptance of TSTG to attack transsexual and transgender people on the basis that the phenomena are pathological. The purpose of these lists is to provide standard codes for insurance claims. As noted earlier, the list compiled by the American Psychiatric Association is the DSM. The international list is the ICD, and it covers all diseases as well as mental disorders. In the United States, the ICD is compliant with the Health Insurance Portability and Accountability Act and is recognized by the federal government as the only list to be used for billing purposes. The DSM is used extensively in the United States and other countries, but since 2003, its codes must be converted to ICD codes for billing purposes. The process of setting up the conversion process is guided by a "harmonization" of the DSM and ICD, which sets up pointers for conversion from DSM to ICD codes.

In 2013, with some fanfare, the fifth version of the DSM (DSM-V) was released with reports that TSTG had been depathologized by virtue of the establishment of a separate category for "gender dysphoria" and a few other changes. This depathologization turned out to be disappointing for several reasons.

For one thing, although gender dysphoria is a separate chapter of the DSM-V it is still in the DSM, which is supposed to be a listing of mental disorders. The last word in the DSM title is still "disorder." In comparison, depathologization of homosexuality in 1973 involved total deletion of homosexuality from the DSM. Supporters of establishment of the gender dysphoria code argue that the DSM has to contain some code to allow for treatment of TSTG people, including TS GPS. This argument is weak because most TSTG will not be diagnosed with "gender dysphoria" for insurance purposes, just as few people were diagnosed with gender identity disorder in the past. There are plenty of other codes that were and are currently used to counsel TSTG people because they carry less stigma. A code to justify TS GPS is the only remaining problem. One of the reasons it remains a problem in the United States is that Medicare now covers TS GPS, and presumably Medicare would require a code that justifies TS GPS. The easiest way to deal with these problems is to change the title of the DSM to allow for inclusion of nonpathological mental phenomena that nevertheless need treatment.

Second, as noted earlier, ICD-9 is used in the United States for billing purposes. With regard to codes pertinent to TSTG, ICD-9 has no "gender dysphoria" category and resembles DSM-IV more closely that DSM-V. The DSM-V and ICD-10 have not been "harmonized," but it is clear that there is not a pointer to a "gender dysphoria" code in the ICD-10. This indicates that the new "gender dysphoria" code is meaningless with regard to billing through the ICD-10 and that ICD will continue its pathologization of TSTG. It is believed that in the next version of the ICD (ICD-11), TSTG will be "depathologized," but that new version is not expected until 2017.

Third, although a code for "gender dysphoria" was added to the DSM-V, several codes that pathologize TSTG continue from the DSM-IV. The most egregious of these is the continuation of autogynephilia into DSM-V. WPATH objected to inclusion of autogynephilia in DSM-V because the "theory" of autogynephilia was unproven. This is consistent with the conclusions of Section 12.1.1.1 in the present volume.

12.3 DEPRESSION

No doubt some transsexuals and transgender people suffer from depression, but their depression does not provide the basis for their TSTG. A recent study of TSTG in Ontario, Canada, estimates that the frequency of major depression in transsexuals and transgender people is 61.2% (Rotondi et al., 2011). This is compared with the frequency in the population at large of major depression of only 2%. As discussed in Chapter 2, TSTG depression appears to be due to secrecy, isolation, and loneliness brought on by rejection from families, communities, and the culture at large. In the Ontario study, depression was also correlated with living outside a big city (Toronto). Big cities can provide more safety, social outlets, resources, and networking for TSTG than rural areas. Of the TSTG who lived outside of Toronto, 72.3% experienced sexual or parental abuse. Unemployment contributed to depression, with only 37.8 employed full time and 40.4% falling in the bottom 10% of income in the country.

Depression has been associated with TSTG around the world—in the United States (Clements-Noelle, Marx, & Katz, 2006), in Hong Kong (Lam et al., 2004), in Switzerland (Hepp et al., 2005), in the Pacific Islands (Operario & Nemoto, 2005), and in Australia/New Zealand (Couch et al., 2007).

Because of the severe life events that transsexuals and transgender people often face, the depression they experience could be classified as reactive depression. Their depression is not due to malfunction of brain mechanisms such as an imbalance of monoamines. Indeed, their depression is a normal human response to a hostile environment that provokes their stress.

In a study of 167 transsexual patients, some who were undergoing hormone therapy (HT), the HT drug treatment clearly helped transsexuals deal with depression (Gómez-Gil et al., 2012). Whether the HT effect is physiological or psychological is undetermined. The antidepressant lithium has been tried in low doses (Coleman & Cesnik, 1990) on a few patients, but antidepressants are not routinely prescribed for TSTG depression. Depression is a result of TSTG, not the cause.

12.4 SUMMARY

Because TSTG is known to be a naturally occurring, benign behavioral phenomenon—a conclusion supported by historical, cultural, and biopsychological evidence (Decker & Pol, 1989; Witten et al., 2003)—it should not be considered an illness or disorder and should not be deliberately or inadvertently pathologized by mental health professionals or by the media. Transsexuals and transgender people sometimes need to seek mental health services for support and, for some, to follow the WPATH guidelines for treatment. The guidelines were created specifically to rule out mental illness and mental incompetence in dealing with treatment or potential transsexual transition decisions.

REFERENCES

American Psychiatric Association. (2013). *Diagnostic and Statistical Manual of Mental Disorders* (5th ed.). Arlington, VA: American Psychiatric Association.

Benjamin, H. (1966). The transsexual phenomenon; a scientific report on transsexualism and sex conversion in the human male and female. Retrieved March 27, 2014, from http://www.mut23.de/texte/Harry%20Benjamin%20-%20The%20Transsexual%20Phenomenon.pdf.

Blanchard, R. (1989). The concept of autogynephilia and the typology of male gender dysphoria. *Journal of Nervous and Mental Disease, 177,* 616–623.

Blanchard, R. (2005). Early history of the concept of autogynephilia. *Archives of Sexual Behavior, 34,* 439–446.

Blanchard, R., Racansky, I., & Steiner, B. (1986). Phallometric detection of fetishistic arousal in heterosexual male cross-dressers. *Journal of Sex Research, 22,* 452–462.

Bodlund, O., Kullgren, G., Sundbom, E., & Hojerback, T. (1993). Personality traits and disorders among transsexuals. *Acta Psychiatrica Scandinavica, 88,* 322–327.

Bruner, J., Goodnow, J., & Austin, G. (1967). *A study of thinking.* New York: Science Editions.

Buhrich, N. (1978). Motivation for cross-dressing in heterosexual transvestism. *Acta Psychiatrica Scandinavica, 57,* 145–152.

Clements-Nolle, K., Marx, R., & Katz, M. (2006). Attempted suicide among transgender persons: The influence of gender-based discrimination and victimization. *Journal of Homosexuality, 51,* 53–69.

Cohen, L., Ruiter, C., Ringelberg, H., & Cohen-Kettenis, P. (1997). Psychological functioning of adolescent transsexuals: Personality and psychopathology. *Journal of Clinical Psychology, 53,* 187–196.

Coleman, E., & Cesnik, J. (1990). Skoptic syndrome: The treatment of an obsessional gender dysphoria with lithium carbonate and psychotherapy. *American Journal of Psychotherapy, 44,* 204–217.

Couch, M., Pitts, M., Mulcare, H., Croy, S., Mitchell, A., & Patel, S. (2007). *Tranznation. A report on the health and wellbeing of transgender people in Australia and New Zealand* (Monograph Series, no. 65). Australian Research Centre in Sex, Health & Society.

Decker, R., & Pol, L. (1989). *The tradition of female transvestism in early modern Europe.* New York: St. Martin's Press.

Devor, H. (1994). Transsexualism, dissociation and child abuse. *Journal of Psychology and Human Sexuality, 6,* 49–72.

Ekins, R., & King, D. (2001, July). Transgendering, migrating and love of oneself as a woman: A contribution to a sociology of autogynephilia. *International Journal of Transgenderism, 5.* Retrieved February 12, 2014, from http://www.iiav.nl/ezines/web/ijt/97-03/numbers/symposion/ijtvo05no03_01.htm.

Feighner, J., Robins, E., Guze, S., Woodruff, R., Winocur, G., & Munoz, R. (1972). Diagnostic criteria for use in psychiatric research. *Archives of General Psychiatry, 26,* 57–63.

Freud, S. (1977). *The origins of psycho-analysis: Letters to Wilhelm Fliess, Drafts and Notes: 1887–1902.* New York: Basic Books. (Original work published 1950.)

Garb, H., Wood, J., Lilienfeld, S., & Nezworski, M. (2005). Roots of the Rorschach controversy. *Clinical Psychology Review, 25,* 97–118.

Gómez-Gil, E., Zubiaurre-Elorza, L., Esteva, I., Guillamon, A., Godás, T., Cruz Almaraz, M., . . . Salamero, M. (2012). Hormone-treated transsexuals report less social distress, anxiety and depression. *Psychoneuroendo, 37,* 662–670.

Hamer, D., Hu, N., Hu, S., Magnusone, V., & Pattatuchi, A. (1993). A linkage between DNA markers on the X chromosome and male sexual orientation. *Science, 261*, 321–327.

Haraldsen, I., & Dahl, A. (2000). Symptom profiles of gender dysphoric patients of transsexual type compared to patients with personality disorders and healthy adults. *Acta Psychiatrica Scandinavica, 102*, 276–281.

Hepp, U., Kraemer, B., Schnyder, U., Miller, N., & Delsignore, A. (2005). Psychiatric comorbidity in gender identity disorder. *Journal of Psychosomatic Research, 58*, 259–261.

Hu, S., Pattatucci, A. M., Patterson, C., Li, L., Fulker, D. W., Cherny, S. S., . . . Hamer, D. H. (1995). Linkage between sexual orientation and chromosome Xq28 in males but not in females. *Nature Genetics, 11*, 248–256.

Kelly, A. (2002). *The psychology of secrets.* New York: Springer.

Kernberg, O. (1977). The structural diagnosis of borderline personality organization. In P. Hartolcollis (Ed.), *Borderline personality disorders.* New York: International Universities Press.

Kersting, A., Reutemann, M., Gast, U., Ohrmann, P., Suslow, T., Michael, N., & Arolt, V. (2003). Dissociative disorders and traumatic childhood experiences in transsexuals. *Journal of Nervous and Mental Disease, 191*, 182–189.

Kruglyak, L., & Lander, E. (1995). Complete multipoint sib-pair analysis of qualitative and quantitative traits. *American Journal of Human Genetics, 57*, 439–454.

Lam, T., Stewart, S. M., Leung, G. M., Lee, P. W., Wong, J. P., Ho, L. M., & the Youth Sexuality Task Force. (2004). Depressive symptoms among Hong Kong adolescents; relation to atypical sexual feelings and behaviors, gender dissatisfaction, pubertal timing, and family and peer relationships. *Archives of Sexual Behavior, 33*, 487–496.

Lawrence, A. (2007). Becoming what we love: Autogynephilic transsexualism conceptualized as an expression of romantic love. *Perspectives in Biology and Medicine, 50*, 506–521.

Lawrence, A. (2006). Clinical and theoretical parallels between desire for limb amputation and gender identity disorder. *Archives of Sexual Behavior, 35*, 263–278.

Lawrence, A. (2003). Factors associated with satisfaction or regret following male-to-female. *Archives of Sexual Behavior 32*, 299–315.

Lilienfeld, S., Wood, J., & Garb, H. (2000). The scientific status of projective techniques. *Psychological Science in the Public Interest, 1*, 27–66.

Lothstein, L. (1979). Group therapy with gender dysphoria patients. *American Journal of Psychotherapy, 333*, 67–81.

Michel, A., & Mormont, C. (2004). Flight into the imaginary world and dependence: Personality trait or opportunist defence mechanism in the transsexual [in French]. *Encephale, 30*, 147–152.

Michel, A., & Mormont, C. (2002). Was Snow White a transsexual [in French]? *Encephale.* 28, 59–64.

Moser, C. (2010). Blanchard's autogynephilia theory: A critique. *Journal of Homosexuality, 57,* 790–809.

Murray, J. (1985). Borderline manifestations in the Rorschachs of male transsexuals. *Journal of Personality Assessment, 49,* 454–466.

Mustanski, B., DuPree, M., Nievergelt, C., Bocklandt, S., Schork, N., & Hamer, D. (2005). Genome wide scan of male sexual orientation. *Human Genetics, 116,* 272–278.

Operario, D., & Nemoto, T. (2005). Sexual risk behavior and substance use among a sample of Asian Pacific Islander transgendered women. *AIDS Education and Prevention, 17,* 430–433.

Rice, W., Friberg, U., & Gavrilets, S. (2012). Homosexuality as a consequence of epigenetically canalized sexual development. *The Quarterly Review of Biology, 87,* 342–368.

Rotondi, N., Bauer, G. R., Travers, R., Travers, A., Scanlon, K., & Kaay, M. (2011). Depression in male-to-female transgender Ontarians: Results from the trans PULSE project. *Canadian Journal of Community Mental Health, 30,* 113–133.

Saks, B. (1998). Transgenderism and dissociative identity disorder—A case study. *International Journal of Transgenderism, 2.* Retrieved February 12, 2014, from http://www.iiav.nl/ezines/web/ijt/97-03/numbers/symposion/ijtc0404.htm.

Socarides, C. (1970). A psychoanalytic study of the desire for sexual transformation ("transsexualism"): The plaster-of-paris man. *International Journal of Psychoanalysis, 51,* 341–349.

Stoller, R. (1968). *Sex and gender.* New York: Science House.

Turner, W. (1995). Homosexuality, type 1: an Xq28 phenomenon. *Archives of Sexual Behavior, 24,* 109–134.

Veale, J. (2005). *Love of oneself as a woman: An investigation into the sexuality of transsexual and other women.* Masters thesis, Massey University, Albany, New York.

Veale, J. F., Lomax, T. C., Clarke, D. E. (2010). The identity-defense model of gender-variant development. *International Journal of Transgenderism, 12*(3), 125–138.

Wailing, D. P., Goodwin, J. M., & Cole, C. M. (1998). Dissociation in a transsexual population. *Journal of Sex Education & Therapy, 23,* 121–123.

Wassersug, R., Zeleniectz, S., & Squire, G. (2004). New age eunuchs: Motivation and rationale for voluntary castration. *Archives of Sexual Behavior, 33,* 433–442.

Winnicott, D. (1971). *Therapeutic consultation in child psychiatry.* London: Hogarth.

Witten, T., Benestad, E. E. P., Berger, I., Elkins, R. J. M., Ettner, R., Harima, K., . . . Sharpe, A. N. (2003). *Transgender and transsexuality.* Academia.

edu. Retrieved March 15, 2014, from http://www.academia.edu/280714/ Transgender_and_Transsexuality

Wood, J. M., Lilienfeld, S., Garb, H., & Nezworski, M. (2000). The Rorschach test in clinical diagnosis: A critical review, with a backward look at Gar-field (1947). *Journal of Clinical Psychology, 56*, 395–430.

Wood, J., Lilienfeld, S. O., Nezworski, M. T., Garb, H. N., Allen, K. H., & Wildermuth, J. L. (2010). Validity of Rorschach inkblot scores for discriminating psychopaths from non-psychopaths in forensic population: A meta-analysis. *Psychological Assessments, 22*, 336–349.

Wood, J. M., Nezworski, M., Lilienfeld, S., & Garb, H. (2003). *What's wrong with the Rorschach? Science confronts the controversial inkblot test.* New York: Jossey-Bass.

Wood, J. M., Nezworski, M. T., Garb, H. N., & Lilienfeld, S. O. (2001a). The misperception of psychopathology: Problems with the norms of the Comprehensive System for the Rorschach. Clinical Psychology: Science and Practice, 8, 350–373.

Wood, J. M., Nezworski, M. T., Garb, Howard, N., & Lilienfeld, S. O. (2001b) Problems with the norms of the Comprehensive System for the Rorschach: Methodological and conceptual considerations. Clinical Psychology: Science and Practice, 8, 397–402

Transition Procedures and Outcomes

13.0 INTRODUCTION

There seems to be intense curiosity about transsexual transition. Since Christine Jorgensen came out in the early 1950s, the idea of "changing sexes" has captured more interest than the phenomenon of transsexualism and transgenderism (TSTG) itself. This curiosity is often seen in media interviews of transsexuals in which the interviewer focuses on surgical changes to genitalia. Transsexuals are often pigeonholed into those preoperative and postoperative for transsexual genital plastic surgery (GPS). For some only postop transsexuals are considered "real" transsexuals, but this is a mistaken notion. This chapter describes the procedures involved with both male-to-female (MTF) and female-to-male (FTM) transition.

There are many misconceptions about transsexual transition. Although medical science and surgical technique have advanced to the point where external sex organs can resemble the opposite sex, especially for MTF, "sex changes" are not complete. Future advances in surgical technique, uterine transplants, organ transplants, and gene therapy may improve the ability of transsexuals to come closer to actually changing sex.

Another misconception is that transition is like some sort of mountain climbing expedition in which transsexuals fail if they do not reach the summit, defined as completing transsexual GPS. Transition is an individual matter in which transsexuals take it one step at a time. At each step, they make a separate decision whether to take a next step in body change based on their feelings of congruence with the sex associated with their congruent gender behavior category. In fact, only a small proportion of transsexuals actually undergo transsexual GPS (Futterweit, 1998).

A third misconception is that only transsexuals undergo the procedures included in transsexual transition. Some nontranssexual transgender people also undergo some of these procedures. For example, many nontranssexual transgender people experiment with hormones on a do-it-yourself basis and many even get breast implants. The hormones involved can be obtained in many countries without prescription. This experimentation with hormones sometimes makes it difficult to establish whether supposed pre–hormone therapy (HT) transsexuals have indeed not taken hormones previously. So describing transition procedures helps in understanding both transgenderism and transsexualism behavior.

Mental and medical health professionals generally follow established professional guidelines for transsexual transition. The international professional guideline-setting organization is the World Professional Association for Transgender Health (WPATH, 2013). There are other important guidelines such as those published by the Endocrine Society (Hembree et al., 2009) for HT, guidelines from the Royal College of Psychiatrists (1988), and treatment guidelines from the American College of Obstetrics and Gynecology (2011). Individual countries and provinces also have their own guidelines, although they generally follow WPATH but also provide local procedures for treatment. The Canadian Professional Association for Transgender Health (2014) offers an online course for endocrine treatment guidelines for Canadian transsexual transition. A list of guideline sources is included in Appendix B.

Many transsexuals and transgender people do not always seek out mental health professionals to follow the appropriate guidelines. This is especially true for nontranssexual transgender people. Transgender people are reluctant to seek mental health treatment for many reasons (Shipherd, Green, & Abrawovitz, 2010) but especially to avoid social stigma. There are many do-it-yourself sources of information including how to buy hormones from pharmacies in countries where no prescriptions are required. Breast implants and even transsexual GPS can be obtained from surgeons who do not follow professional guidelines requiring recommendation letters for surgery. The medical risks of transition procedures are increased for unsupervised transition. Do-it-yourself HT can result in both overdosing due to lack of blood test monitoring and underdosing due to counterfeit drugs.

Transition procedures can complicate medical treatment of transsexuals and transgender people. When giving their own medical histories, some transsexuals and transgender people may be reluctant to admit that they are taking hormones or that they may have had other transition procedures. This includes transsexual GPS because surgical results are frequently so good that they are indistinguishable from natal genitalia, particularly for MTF. Postop transsexuals who are living in secrecy or "stealth mode" may avoid giving complete medical histories to medical personnel in the presence of family members so as not to arouse suspicion about their past. Most transsexuals and transgender people know that the Hippocratic oath is supposed to protect their medical histories, but there are notorious examples of violations of the oath. There are also examples of medical personnel refusing to render treatment if a person's TSTG status is known. This has included microaggressions such as mockery of the patient by medical health professionals as well as refusal to provide prescribed medicines. In this day of digital medical health records, it is quite possible for unauthorized people to view the records of transsexuals despite the best computer security.

Few mental health professionals are expert in supervision of transsexual transition, and it is important that those contemplating transition find one or more of these experts. Both medical school and mental health training curricula do not cover TSTG in any detail, and it is not a recognized professional specialty. Because TSTG is not an illness or disorder, the job of a mental health professional primarily consists of providing counseling for dealing with interpersonal issues and patient management. Patient management involves such mundane things as guidance on where one can get suitably sized clothing, which public accommodations are safe, where to find an understanding hairdresser, and which surgeons are reliable. Thus, patient management requires knowledge of the local and national TSTG community and subculture.

The goal of transition is to make sex organs look more male or more female and help bring TSTG presentation into alignment with cultural expectations of a person's congruent gender behavior category of a transsexual. However, the needs of each transsexual are different. WPATH and other transition guidelines are flexible and can be tailored to each transsexual. For example, some MTF transsexuals do not receive HT but instead jump directly to breast enlargement. The results of previous transition events need to be continuously evaluated by the transsexual and a mental health professional to determine whether any additional procedures are needed and what they should be.

The philosophy of transition emphasizes the minimization of potential harm. Transition usually starts with those procedures that are nearly completely reversible, such as taking blocking agents that suppress puberty in children or hormone therapy. As described in Chapter 8, such blocking agents are especially useful for treating children who want to avoid puberty or at least delay it until they can decide whether to start transsexual transition. The other nearly reversible procedures are HT that result in MTF breast growth and infertility in FTM. MTF breast growth due to HT can be reversed surgically, and FTM infertility can be reversed by stopping HT.

Next, procedures that have irreversible consequences are undertaken. These are primarily surgical procedures such as breast enhancement, facial feminization surgery (FFS), and transsexual GPS for MTF. These typically occur after HT is well under way. Breast reduction for FTM can start at the beginning of HT. Transsexual GPS is usually delayed until successful full-time real-life experience (RLE) in the new gender behavior category has been successfuly completed.

13.1 THE MOTIVATION FOR TRANSITION PROCEDURES

The motivation to bring one's gender presentation into congruence with cultural expectations of one's congruent gender behavior category can increase the urgency for transsexuals and transgender people to alter their bodies. For some transgender people, occasional or regular cross-dressing may not suffice, although it may bring temporary relief and relaxation (Buhrich, 1978). As we saw in Chapter 11, the motivation for TSTG is mediated by subconscious mechanisms that cannot be directly controlled by conscious thought. This is true for all human motivation and decisions, not just those of people with TSTG. Other subconscious mechanisms may represent the competition between the drive for TSTG behavior and other factors including family, friends, and making a living. Chapter 11 also described how an existential crisis can promote TSTG behavior and increase its frequency or the motivation for transition.

Transsexual transition usually has positive results. Undergoing transition procedures reduces suffering from incongruence and reduces depression. In a survey of adolescents, 90% report reduced incongruence (Close, 2012) that continued during HT and transsexual GPS.

Also at play is the need for authenticity. Transsexual and transgender people may go through a period of cross-dressing or living in which they resort to wearing false breasts, wigs, heavy makeup, breast binding, and padded clothes. Such artificiality becomes a time and resource burden and seems like a waste of time. At some point, especially when they get tired of their fling at artificiality, the drive for authenticity leads some to want their bodies to be authentic and match their gender predisposition.

For some transsexuals and transgender people, attractiveness in presentation is important and, in particular, breast realism and size become a priority. Although transgender people can create the illusion of natural breasts or even cleavage with breast forms and makeup, it can become burdensome and time-consuming. It should be no surprise that males perceive breast size as important in attractiveness (Zelazniewicz & Pawlowski, 2011), and if a transsexual or transgender person is attracted to males, breast enhancement becomes a priority. Attractiveness and authenticity also helps transsexuals and transgender people to pass in public, which has practical benefits of reducing harassment and violence.

Expert mental health professionals try to encourage transsexual and transgender people to present in their preferred gender behavior category for increasingly longer periods of time. TSTG conventions, gatherings, and cruises provide opportunities for longer presentation periods in a safe environment. The longer periods serve several purposes. They provide transsexuals and transgender people with longer periods of relief and relaxation from their incongruent assigned gender behavior category and to perfect their presentation in the gender behavior category in which they might want to live. These longer periods provide opportunities for flooding desensitization that reduces the sexual arousal associated with cross-dressing and TSTG behavior. This allows transsexuals and transgender people to experience their preferred gender behavior category with lower sexual arousal. It allows the mental health professional to determine whether TSTG behavior continues with reduced sexual arousal. Longer periods also constitute behavior rehearsals for transsexualism for a future time in which they might undergo the procedure of RLE.

Surveys show that transition improves the quality of life for transsexuals and results in reduced depression and improved quality of life. As we saw in Chapter 12, the depression experienced by transsexuals and transgender people is usually situational or reactive depression brought on by conflicts with culture. These longer periods of living in the gender behavior category that fits them best provide opportunities for transsexuals and transgender people to experience alleviation of depression and improved quality of life. Reports of these experiences help the mental health professional confirm that the depression experienced by transsexuals and transgender people is situational and not due to an underlying organic depression.

13.2 TRANSITION PROCEDURES

Obviously, transition procedures differ between MTF and FTM, although the philosophy of approach is similar. The general philosophy is that reversible procedures should be undertaken early in the process with irreversible procedures reserved for the end of the transition process. This allows a transsexual and their mental health and medical health teams to continuously evaluate whether they want to proceed further.

13.2.1 MTF Transition Procedures

There are nine categories of MTF transition procedures as follows:

- Mental health assessment
- HT

- Facial hair removal
- Hair regrowth
- Breast implants
- Facial feminization surgery
- Real-life experience
- Transsexual GPS
- Voice therapy

Each of these are discussed in turn in the following sections.

13.2.1.1 MTF Mental Health Assessment

Referral letters from mental health professionals are needed for several MTF transition procedures under the WPATH guidelines, particularly feminization HT and surgeries. Two letters are required for transsexual genital surgery. The letters are only provided after a thorough assessment and after offering supportive care and patient management services. The supportive care may extend to family and significant others. Psychotherapy is not a requirement for transition procedures. The assessment includes exploration of any co-occurring mental health issues. The procedure also includes providing information about possible transition procedures.

WPATH criteria for referral letters include the following:

1. Persistent, well-documented gender dysphoria;
2. Capacity to make a fully informed decision and to consent for treatment.
3. Age of majority in a given country; . . .
4. If significant medical or mental health concerns are present, they must be reasonably controlled. (WPATH, 2013)

With reference to the third criteria, WPATH has additional requirements for transsexuals and transgender people who are not of majority that were discussed in Chapters 8 and 9.

For surgeries, the WPATH criteria includes:

12 continuous months of hormone therapy as appropriate to the patient's gender goals unless hormones are not clinically indicated for the individual. (WPATH, 2013)

Because assessment for transition procedures requires information from the prospective transsexual, there is concern that the patient is essentially providing a self-diagnosis. The expert TSTG mental health professional is usually able to see through patients' attempts to manipulate their assessment.

Before HT is started, MTF transsexuals should develop a transition plan with their mental health professional. This should feature a social transition plan. How will the transsexual dress and comport themselves during HT and beyond? Who will provide social support for the transsexual during transition?

13.2.1.2 MTF HT

HT is sometimes referred to as *hormone replacement therapy* or HRT, but the correct term, according to WPATH, is simply hormone therapy (HT). In most all cases, hormones are given for TSTG not to replace hormones previously lost by age or accident but to induce body change. A referral letter to an endocrinologist or physician is usual to begin HT. It is best if the medical professional has experience with transsexual transition. The goals of HT are to induce cross-sex secondary sex characteristics while reducing or eliminated the effects of endogenous sex hormones (Olson, 2012).

Table 13.1 shows a menu of drugs and nominal dosages that might be used in MTF HT. The information in this table comes from the Endocrine Society Guidelines (Hembree et al., 2009) with updates by WPATH (WPATH, 2013) and unique information from treating homeless and poor transsexuals from other sources (Burnett, 2011a, 2011b; Davidson et al., 2013; Olson, 2012).

Drugs, selection, dosage, and route of administration vary by physician and individual transsexual situation and body weight. All of these drugs in Table 13.1 are prescribed off-label with respect to the U.S. Food and Drug Administration. There are several recommended baseline protocols with variations. Some physicians prefer to use injected or implanted drugs, particularly for patients who are in poverty or on the street. These routes of administration are used because they require less patient responsibility and because patients must come in regularly, facilitating examinations and testing for venereal diseases and HIV.

Oral estradiol blocks release of hypothalamic gonadotropin-releasing hormone (GnRH) that normally stimulates release of testosterone through other hormones. Release of GnRH in the hypothalamus causes release of luteinizing and follicle-stimulating hormones in the pituitary. This, in turn, triggers synthesis and release of testosterone from the testes. Excessive testosterone feeds back on the GnRH mechanism in the hypothalamus and reduces the testosterone level. The GnRH feedback mechanism responds, not only to testosterone but also estradiol and progesterone.

Estradiol feminizes the body and stimulates grown of *stromal* tissue in the breast that determines breast structure. Combined with progesterone, estradiol also develops a second type of tissue, the *lobular* tissue of the breast, which is the actual milk-secreting tissue. In HT, the dosage of oral estradiol should be minimized because the most severe adverse side effects of MTF HT

Table 13.1. Drugs and nominal dosages for male-to-female hormone therapy

Drug	Route of Administration	Nominal Dosages	Interval	Protocol
Estradiol valerate	Oral	2–6 mg	Daily	SYPP; Gooren
Estradiol ethinyl		Not used		
Estradiol	Sublingual	1–4 mg	Daily	UCSF
Estradiol	Transdermal	100–400 mcg	Daily	UCSF; SYPP
Estradiol valerate	Intramuscular	5–20 mg	Biweekly	UCSF; SYPP
Estradiol valerate	Intramuscular	40 mg	Biweekly	Burnett b
Spironolactone	Oral	100–400 mg	Daily	UCSF
Ciproterone	Oral	100 mg	Daily	Gooren
Goserlin	Oral	UNK		
Buserelin	Oral	UNK		
Triptorelin	Oral	UNK		
Finasteride	Oral	2.5–5 mg	Daily	UCSF; SYPP
Dutasterone	Oral	UNK	Daily	UCSF-Burnett b
Methylprogesterone	Oral	5–10 mg	Daily	UCSF-Burnett b
Depo medoxyprogesterone	Intramuscular	150 mg	3 months	SYPP-Olson
Prometrium	Oral	100–200 mg	Daily	UCSF-Burnett b
Depo-Provera progesterone Viagra	Intramuscular	150mg	3 Months	UCSF-Burnett b
Depo Provera (illicit use)	Oral	UNK		UCSF-Burnett a
Depo Provera (illicit use)	Intramuscular	UNK		UCSF-Burnett a
Perlutal (illicit use)	Oral	UNK		UCSF-Burnett a
Perlutal (illicit use)	Intramuscular	UNK		UCSF-Burnett a
Phytoestrogens	Oral	UNK		UCSF-Burnett a

are believed to result from estrogens (see Section 13.2.1.2.2). Estrogen also increases the levels of sex hormone–binding globulin (SHBG), which binds to testosterone and inactivates it. Estrogen also seems to maintain sexual interest even when testosterone levels are minimized (Wibowo, Schelltammer, & Wassersug 2011).

Testosterone blocking agents are usually used to minimize the dosage of estradiol needed. Spironolactone blocks both testosterone release and blocks testosterone receptors that transmit messages to body cells. However, spirono-lactone is also an antihypertensive and potassium-sparing drug that results in lower blood pressure. For this reason, blood pressure and potassium levels should be monitored if it is prescribed. Spironolactone also reduces libido and arrests male pattern baldness. In Europe and some parts of the world, cyproterone is used in place of spironolactone, but it is not generally used in the United States because of potential side effects on liver function. Cyproter-one also has progestinergic effects, so levels of progesterone should be moni-tored, and interactions with the possible administration of progesterone in HT should be monitored.

Sex hormone blockers similar to those used to block puberty (described in Section 8.4.2; goserelin, buserelin, and triptorelin) are sometimes also pre-scribed in MTF HT. Their action is to minimize synthesis and release of tes-tosterone by reducing GnRH release. These drugs are rarely prescribed for MTF HT because they are expensive and GnRH release can usually be sup-pressed by estrogen and progesterone alone.

The synthesis blockers finasteride (Propecia) and dutasteride prevent the synthesis of dihydrotestosterone (DHT) from testosterone. DHT is a highly active version of testosterone that masculinizes the body during normal development. These synthesis blockers are particularly useful in reducing the effects of any remaining testosterone in the body and in reducing male pat-tern baldness.

Progestins, usually in the form of medroxyprogesterone, are administered as part of HT to decrease GnRH release, which in turn reduces synthesis and release of testosterone from the testes. Progestins also stimulate the growth of lobular breast tissue that estradiol by itself does not influence to optimize breast development. There are suspicions that progestins have unwanted side effects (breast cancer risk, cardiovascular risk, depression, and weight gain). In particular, there is intense research on the interactions of estrogens and progestins in postmenopausal women that might trigger certain forms of breast cancer. The risks of taking progestins should be weighed against the risks of breast enhancement surgery, which are not inconsiderable.

Illicit drugs are often used by transsexuals and transgender people to avoid dealing with a physician. They are mentioned here to help understand that the need for voluntary body change by TSTG is urgent and is pursued even through illegal channels. Physicians need to be aware that such drugs are in circulation. Although drug importation is banned by the United States, the drugs estradiol, progesterone, and spironolactone are readily available from offshore pharmacies on the Internet. No prescription is necessary. A common drug that is obtained illicitly is Depo-Provera, or medroxyproges-terone. It is used primarily for birth control, but chemical variations also used illicitly for MTF HT in the United States. Under the brand name Perlutal, it is smuggled across the Mexico–United States border and used illicitly for MTF HT in poor Hispanic communities in southern California (Burnett, 2011b). It consists of a derivative of estradiol and a progestin drug, either algestone acetophenide or a derivative of algestone depending on the country of origin. Manufacture of these derivatives may be an attempt to avoid patent infringement, and little is known about them scientifically. Perlutol is a formulary used primarily in Colombia, Mexico, and Peru as a contraceptive.

It is important also to know that illicit drugs are sometimes counterfeit because they are uncontrolled. Drugs from the same pharmacy can vary in potency. This can result in wide swings in actual dosage and effects. It is important that transsexuals and transgender people avoid illicit drugs.

Phytoestrogens are sometimes used by transsexuals and transgender people without medical supervision. They have mild estrogenic effects but are not as effective as prescribed estrogens. Large quantities of these drugs are needed to provide an effect and at those doses phytoestrogens are toxic.

13.2.1.2.1 Effects of MTF HT

Some of the known effects of MTF HT are listed in Table 13.2. The information in this table is from the Endocrine Society Guidelines (Hembree et al., 2009) with updates by the Canadian Professional Association for Transgender Health (2014) and WPATH (2011) and contributions from other sources (Burnett, 2011a; 2011b; Davidson et al., 2013; Olson, 2012).

Although the height and overall structure of the body does not change during MTF HT, there are significant changes to muscle, fat distribution, and skin and hair growth. The MTF transsexual loses muscle mass and strength, which is one of the rationales that MTF transsexuals should be allowed to compete athletically as a female. Body fat is gradually distributed to female proportions. Skin becomes soft and dry, requiring constant moisturization. Body and facial hair become thin and brittle, which assists in removal.

Because testosterone production and release is no longer stimulated by the hypothalamus to the gonads, the only testosterone source remaining is the adrenal glands. With some HT drug protocols, testosterone production is slowed by synthesis blockers and receptor blockers. Libido becomes reduced, as does spontaneous erection. Eventually testicular volume becomes reduced and nonpermanent testicular shrinkage occurs. Ejaculate decreased in sperm concentration until fertility is gone. For this reason, many MTF transsexuals bank their sperm before HT if they want children in the future. Some have successfully restored fertility and loss of libido after long cessation of MTF HT.

Table 13.2. Known effects of male-to-female hormone therapy. CPATH = Canadian Professional Association for Transgender Health; ES = Endocrine Society Guidelines (Hembree et al., 2009); SYPP = Strengthening Youth Prevention Paradigms, Olson, 2012; UCSF = University of California at San Francisco Center of Excellence for Transgender Health (2014); WPATH = World Professional Association for Transgender Health (2013).

Effect	Source
Decreased muscle mass/strength	ES/WPATH
Body fat redistribution to approximate female	ES/WPATH
Accretion of bone-mineral content	UCSF-Burnett
Softening of skin/dry skin	ES/WPATH
Thinning and slowed growth of body and facial hair	ES/WPATH
Decreased libido/difficulty reaching orgasm	CPATH
Male sexual dysfunction	ES/WPATH
Decreased spontaneous/morning erections	CPATH
Progressive reduction in testicular volume to 50%	CPATH
Nonpermanent testicular shrinkage	UCSF-Burnett
Infertility	SYPP
Tender breast buds within 3–6 months	CPATH
Breast and nipple growth through 2 years	CPATH
Permanent changes to nipple-areolae	CPATH
Heightened sense of touch	SYPP-Olson
Increased sense of smell	SYPP-Olson
Increased emotionality	SYPP-Olson
Will not raise voice pitch	UCSF-Burnett
Will not shrink Adam's apple	UCSF-Burnett
Will not cause regression of the beard	UCSF-Burnett

Breast growth begins with tender breast buds, and breast and nipple growth continue for at least 2 years just as it does in female puberty. The changes to the breast and nipple/areolae do not go away if HT is withdrawn but can be reversed by surgery.

Attributes usually associated with femininity such as heightened sensory experience and increased emotionality occur. MTF transsexuals report increased spontaneous crying and crying from emotional dramas.

Although all of these changes occur with MTF HT, several changes do not, and this must be explained to the transsexual. For example, MTF HT will not raise voice pitch or feminize voice inflection, so voice therapy may be necessary. The Adam's apple will not shrink, so some MTF transsexuals get surgical reduction, a "tracheal shave," of this neck structure. MTF HT will not stop growth of the facial beard, but it will slow its growth, so facial hair removal is often needed.

13.2.1.2.2 Potential Risks and Side Effects of MTF HT

In general, MTF HT is safe and effective if performed under the supervision of a physician. Table 13.3 shows the potential risks and side effects of MTF hormone therapy. Physicians, transsexuals, and nontranssexual transgender people should be aware of the potential risks and side effects so that they are able to promptly recognize them. This is particularly true for cardiovascular problems (Asscheman et al., 2013; Wierckx et al., 2012). These cardiovascular problems have been reduced in recent years by switching away from ethinyl estradiol to estradiol valerate, but vigilance is still in order. It is important to note that HT transition is not without risk, which indicates the commitment of transsexuals to this procedure to reduce incongruence.

By far the most important increased risk of MTF HT is the potential development of thrombosis or blood clots in veins. Smoking is an additional risk

Table 13.3. Potential risks and side effects of male-to-female hormone therapy. WPATH = World Professional Association for Transgender Health.

Risk	Risk Level Per WPATH
Thrombosis	Likely increased risk
Cardiovascular disease	Likely increased risk with additional factors
Hypertension	Possible increased risk
Hyperprolactinemia or prolactinoma	Possible increased risk
Type 2 diabetes	Possible increased risk with additional risk factors
Gallstones	N/A
Elevated liver enzymes or liver disease	N/A
Weight gain	N/A
Hypertriglyceridemia	N/A

factor in thrombosis, so MTF transsexuals under HT should abstain from smoking. Thrombosis can occur without warning and may result in blockages in circulation, which can result in death. Older studies using ethinyl estradiol HT indicated that 6% to 8% of transsexuals had cardiovascular problems, but this frequency has declined since the use of estradiol valerate began. Estradiol valerate is safer and the estrogen of choice for many doctors (Gooren, Giltay, & Bunck, 2007). Many do-it-yourselfers now use estradiol valerate but frequently overdose, which results in cardiovascular problems (Asscheman et al., 2013). MTF undergoing HT should be particularly alert to symptoms of heart attack or shortness of breath.

Some estrogens are required in almost all MTF HT protocols. Because of the use of estrogen in contraceptives, the mechanisms involved in thrombosis are well established and understood (Tchaikovski & Rosing, 2010). As a result of this research, most medical practitioners minimize the dosage of estrogen by using a combination protocol of testosterone synthesis blockers, receptor blockers, and progesterone.

MTF transsexuals undergoing HT are also at increased risk of several other conditions, but these have slower onset compared with thrombosis and can be detected during regular physicals. These include gallstones, liver disease, weight gain, and high blood triglyceride levels. A MTF may be at even more risk for some of these if additional factors for heart disease are present.

There is a remote risk of high prolactin levels due to a prolactinoma, so WPATH recommends that prolactin levels should be monitored. A prolactinoma is a benign growth near the pituitary that secretes prolactin, a hormone involved in lactation. Prolactin levels can easily be monitored by a blood test. A prolactinoma is treatable using dopamine therapy or surgery.

Although the risk is remote, three MTF transsexuals have been found to have prolactinomas (Garcia-Malpartida, Martin-Gorgojo, Rocha, Gomez-Balaguer, and Hernandez-Mijares, 2010; Gooren, Assies, Asscheman, de Slegte, & van Kessel, 1988; Kovacs, Stefaneanu, Ezzat, & Smyth, 1994). Pituitary swelling with associated high prolactin levels have been found in two MTF transsexuals (Serri, Noiseux, Robert, & Hardy, 1996; Asscheman, 1988). The *sella turcica* is a pocket in the sphenoid bone at the base of the brain that accommodates the pituitary. One study indicated enlargement of the *sella turcica* pocket that might indicate a prolactinoma in posthumous analysis of the skulls of 11 MTF transsexuals (Lundberg, Sjovall, & Walinder, 1975).

Prolactin is regulated in part by estrogen levels (Fink, 1988), and high estrogen levels can produce prolactinomas in humans and animals. In humans, a prolactinoma in one person was associated with exposure to large doses of estrogen from an industrial accident (Baron, Sowers, & Feinberg, 1983). In rats, in has been determined that large doses of estrogen produce prolactinomas (Xu, Wu, Di, Xu, Pang, & Pang, 2000). The mechanisms involved in producing a prolactinoma are unclear. However, prolactinomas occur in .1% of the population (Vroonen, Daly, & Beckers, 2013), so these occurrences in transsexuals could have happened by chance. In any case, prolactinomas can be easily detected with an inexpensive blood test for prolactin (recommended by WPATH and the Endocrine Society for routine examinations). Prolactinomas are also successfully treated with drugs and surgery.

There does not appear to be increased risk of reduced bone density in MTF HT, but Van Caenegem et al. (2013) found that MTF transsexuals already have low bone density before HT begins. No one knows why this would be so. Because bone-density measurement can now be made in a doctor's office using low-cost scanners for hands or legs, it may be prudent for MTF transsexuals starting HT to receive a bone-density scan.

There have not been studies to quantify the overall risks of MTF HT. The objective of most studies on female hormones has been to understand their effects in natal females to address such issues as whether it is safe for postmenopausal women to undergo replacement therapy. However, it appears that, if properly supervised by a qualified physician, the risks of MTF HT are minimal.

13.2.1.2.3 Clinical Monitoring in MTF HT

Both MTF and FTM transsexuals undergoing HT should regularly have physician visits and their relevant blood levels monitored. MTF should be especially examined for cardiovascular disease symptoms. They should be examined for the risks and side effects shown in Table 13.3. Blood level testing should include testosterone, estrogen, progestin, prolactin, potassium (if spironolactone is prescribed), plus tests of general health. Prolactin should especially be measured if pituitary tests indicate potential pressure from a prolactinoma growth. Because the risk for breast cancer is low in MTF, mammograms are needed after 1 year and then only at 10-year intervals. After transsexual GPS, HT may be eliminated or greatly reduced, but monitoring should continue.

13.2.1.3 Facial Hair Removal

Most MTF transsexuals undergo facial hair removal procedures to avoid beard shadow, which is a telltale sign of maleness. Beard shadow is difficult to hide even with the many beard concealer products on the market. Perhaps surprisingly, most of these concealers are bright orange-red and they are applied under makeup.

There are several technologies for beard removal, but the two most common are laser removal or electrolysis. Both technologies attempt to kill off hair follicles through injury. Laser hair removal has been studied for MTF transsexuals and found to be useful (Schroeter, Greenewegen, Beinekier, & Neumann, 2003). Laser removal works best for those with darker hair pigmentation because the laser light is not absorbed as much by blond or gray hair. The yield for laser technology is not as high as for electrolysis, but it is less painful.

Electrolysis involves inserting a fine needle into the hair follicle and transmitting electricity, either direct current or radio current or both, through the needle to coagulate the hair follicle. Electrolysis requires many hours of such treatment because the hair regrowth rate is about 50% even for the most skilled electrologists. Depending on beard density, a MTF may spend several hundred hours to achieve satisfactory results. Electrology is extremely painful, so many MTF get local anesthetics administered by a physician or dentist before their appointments.

13.2.1.4 Hair Regrowth

MTF who begin HT when they are older may have already lost hair due to male pattern balding. For them, there are three choices. They can apply topical minoxidil and Propecia (finasteride) solutions to the affected area; if oral finasteride is used as part of transition, this will help the process of hair restoration. MTF can also get hair transplants. Finally, if the bald area is in the front of the head, they can get a scalp advance operation to reduce the size of the hairless forehead, which brings the hair closer to the front of the head.

13.2.1.5 Breast Implants

Breast growth in MTF HT is only satisfactory about half the time. Despite all attempts to naturally grow breast tissue during HT, the process is not exactly like breast development in the natal female. In particular, growth hormone may be lower in adults than in teenagers. Because of this low satisfaction rate, many MTF transsexuals get breast implants to reshape and increase the size of their breasts. Reshaping is sometimes needed if the breasts develop in a tubular shape or if the breasts are too far apart to look natural.

Getting breast implants is not without risk, although it is getting safer. Older implants broke, spilling their contents. For a while, only saline-filled breast implants were available, but newer silicon and composite technology appears to be safe (U.S. Food and Drug Administration, 2011). Most MTF transsexuals take progesterone as part of HT to improve breast development, which has potential side effects. The risks of taking progesterone should be compared with the risk of side effects from breast implants. Breast implants must still be regarded as temporary because they will have to be removed and replaced in the future.

13.2.1.6 Facial Feminization Surgery

There are now plastic surgeons who specialize in various feminization surgeries for MTF transsexuals and transgender people. The procedures are aimed at reducing male anatomy of the face and neck through scalp advance, rhinoplasty, chin reduction, brow lift, and cheek and lip augmentation. The Adam's apple may be reduced with a "tracheal shave." Feminization surgery can go a long way to help an MTF "pass" as a female.

13.2.1.7 Real-Life Experience

The purpose of the RLE is to gain confidence that the MTF transsexual can live and work as a woman before committing to transsexual GPS. In the RLE, the MTF spends full time presenting as a woman for at least a year. Success of the RLE must be carefully assessed by transsexuals and their mental health professional. WPATH does not require RLE but Many surgeons do.

13.2.1.8 Transsexual GPS

Transsexual GPS is used here to refer to surgery that changes male external genitalia to resemble female genitalia. In transsexual GPS, most penile erectile tissue is removed, and a vagina is created using the remaining tissue from the male genitalia. This can be accomplished in one operation, although some surgeons use a two-step approach to allow healing before final adjustment. Transsexual GPS techniques have greatly improved since the mid-20th century.

For many years, the most prolific transsexual GPS surgeon was Stanley Biber, who conducted his operations in Trinidad, Colorado, but the center of activity now seems to be on the East and West Coast and in Arizona. With more than 1,100 transsexual GPS operations, the current leader in transsexual GPS in the United States appears to be Marci Bowers, but there are other surgeons who are quite competent. She is herself a MTF transsexual who worked with Biber for many years. Transsexual GPS is performed all over the world, but the countries with the highest number are Iran and Thailand, although Serbia is trying to develop its industry (Bilefsky, 2012). Transsexual GPS is frequently done through medical tourism, mainly to Thailand and now also to Serbia.

Complications from MTF transsexual GPS mainly involve urinary tract blockage and infections that are treatable.

13.2.1.9 Voice Therapy

Hormones do not change voice pitch or inflection, so some MTF take voice therapy to sound more like natal females. Fortunately, there is a considerable overlap between natal males and females in the fundamental frequency of their voices. The task of the MTF with regard to pitch is to try to get into that overlapping frequency space. Pitch is not the only difference between natal males and females. Voice inflection, timber, and choice of words and phrases all are different for females but can be learned once the trainee reaches the frequency overlap area. There are several expert voice coaches who specialize in voice change for MTF in person (see Appendix B), and courseware is available on CD.

13.2.2 FTM Transition Procedures

There are seven categories of MTF transition procedures as follows:

- Mental health assessment
- HT
- Mastectomy
- Masculinization surgery
- Real-life experience
- Transsexual GPS
- Voice therapy

Each of these is discussed in turn in the following sections.

13.2.2.1 FTM Mental Health Assessment

Mental health assessment is the same as described in Section 13.2.1.1 for MTF health assessment except that, of course, procedures to increase male appearance are involved in the required referral letters for GPS surgeries.

13.2.2.2 FTM HT

Table 13.4 shows the drugs and nominal dosages involved in FTM HT. The primary drug used in FTM HT is testosterone. The information in this table is derived from Endocrine Society guidelines (Hembree et al., 2009) and a protocol from the Waddell Health Center (Davidson et al., 2013). Testosterone blocks release of GnRH that normally would increase estrogen synthesis and release in the gonads. Testosterone also increases male appearance of the body. As to route of administration, the oral version is less effective in raising testosterone levels and is seldom used. Intramuscular administration is more efficacious and results in less blood-level variation. Testosterone dosage should be the minimum required to produce a satisfactory effect because of potential side effects. Recently, several testosterone products for absorption into the skin have become available, but there is no published literature on

Table 13.4. Drugs used in female-to-male hormone therapy. AX = axillary; IM = intramuscular; TD = transdermal.

Drug	Route of Administration	Nominal Dosages	Interval	Note
Testosterone cypionate	IM	50–100 mg	2 week	Cottonseed oil
Testosterone enathate	IM	200 mg	2 week	Sesame oil
Testosterone propionate	IM	100–200 mg	2 week	
Depo-testosterone	IM	50–200 mg	2 weeks	
Testosterone patch	TD	5 mg	Daily	
Testosterone gel 1%	TD	5 mg	Daily	
Testosterone 1.62%	TD	No published research		
Testosterone axillary	AX	No published research		
Methy testosterone	Oral	Not used		
Finasteride	Oral	Not available		For male pattern baldness
Topical testosterone	Topical	Subtracted from T dose		For clitoris over-enlargement

whether these products are used for HT. Because testosterone tends to cause male pattern baldness, finasteride is sometimes used to block DHT synthesis. Typically the clitoris becomes enlarged and sensitive due to systemic testosterone administration, but FTM transsexuals sometimes also use topical testosterone to stimulate this organ if the systemic approach is insufficient. If so, a decrease in systemic testosterone may be prescribed.

13.2.2.2.1 Effects of FTM HT

In FTM HT, creating a male appearance is the objective to make natal FTM females as much like natal males physically as possible. The effects of FTM HT are shown in Table 13.5. The information in this table is derived from Endocrine Society guidelines (Hembree et al., 2009) and publications of the Waddell Health Center (Davidson et al., 2013). Gross body changes feature increases in muscle mass and strength, and redistribution of fat away from

Table 13.5. Effects of female-to-male hormone therapy

Potential Risk	Source
Increased muscle mass	Tom Waddell Health Center
Increased muscle strength	Tom Waddell Health Center
Redistribution of fat	Tom Waddell Health Center
Beard/body hair growth	Endocrine Society
Permanent voice change	Tom Waddell Health Center
Permanent clitoral enlargement	Tom Waddell Health Center
Increased libido	Tom Waddell Health Center
Increased physical energy	Tom Waddell Health Center
Cessation of menses	Endocrine Society
Vaginal atrophy	Endocrine Society
Male pattern scalp hair loss	Endocrine Society
Protection against osteoporosis	Tom Waddell Health Center

the buttocks and hips to other areas. With increased testosterone, there is increased growth of beard and body hair that are difficult to achieve through cosmetics. There are permanent changes in voice and the size of the clitoris. The fundamental voice frequency becomes deeper. As noted earlier, some FTM transsexuals simulate clitoral size and sensitivity using topical testosterone. Libido and physical energy are also increased.

During FTM HT, both cessation of menses and vaginal atrophy occur, although these effects are somewhat reversible. There are several recorded cases of FTM transsexuals who go off HT long enough to conceive and deliver a child.

With increases in DHT, converted from testosterone, male pattern balding begins, which can be treated with both systemic (finasteride) and topical drugs (minoxidil and finasteride). It can also be addressed with hair implants.

Finally, FTM HT is believed to provide some protection against osteoporosis because of increased testosterone levels. Male osteoporosis is usually due to a decline in testosterone in older people that FTM can avoid.

13.2.2.2.2 Potential FTM HT Risks

In general, FTM HT is safe and effective if performed under the supervision of a physician (Wierckx et al., 2012), but there are important risk factors that must be kept in mind. A list of such risks is shown in Table 13.6. Again, the information in this table is derived from Endocrine Society guidelines (Hembree et al., 2009) and publications of the Waddell Health Center (Davidson et al., 2013). None of these risks are as life threatening as thrombosis in MTF

Table 13.6. Potential risks and side effects of female-to-male hormone therapy. WPATH = World Professional Association for Transgender Health.

Risks	Degree of Risk per WPATH
Increased red cells	Likely increased risk
Weight gain	Likely increased risk
Acne	Likely increased risk
Sleep apnea	Likely increased risk
Elevated liver enzymes	Possible risk
Hyperlipidemia	Possible risk
Cardiovascular disease	Possible risk with additional factors
Hypertension	Possible risk with additional factors
Type 2 diabetes	Possible risk with additional factors
Loss of bone density	No increased risk
Breast cancer	No increased risk
Cervical cancer	No increased risk
Ovarian cancer	No increased risk
Uterine cancer	No increased risk

HT, and all are treatable. There does not appear to be an increased risk of the several kinds of cancer, although they are reported for interest.

Of particular concern to physicians is polycystic ovary syndrome (PCOS), which has been reported to be more frequent in FTM transsexuals, although it is often overlooked by physicians who are not expert in FTM transition. This is a relatively common genetic disease (5%–10%) among natal females (Futterweit, 1999). FTM are more likely to exhibit PCOS (Baba et al., 2007; Futterweit & Deligdisch, 1986; Pache & Fauser, 1993). PCOS can be missed in postop FTM transsexuals. PCOS was found in 58% of FTM transsexuals before HT and transsexual GPS (Baba et al., 2007). This is higher than the normal population frequency, although a matched population study has not been done. PCOS was associated with obesity and elevated testosterone levels, although it was suspected in the Baba et al. study (2007) that some FTM transsexuals were self-administering testosterone. Pache and Fauser (1993) believed that elevated androgen levels induce PCOS through follicular mechanisms, regardless of FTM status. In a later study with more rigorous criteria of PCOS using transvaginal ultrasound, no direct relationship was found between PCOS and pre-HT FTM transsexuals compared with control subjects (Mueller et al., 2008). In this study, FTM transsexuals did have elevated levels of testosterone, which may have contributed to PCOS, but 20% of the control subjects with PCOS also had elevated testosterone levels. Although the FTM transsexuals who admitted to previously taking self-administered testosterone were eliminated, the subjects could have misreported this important fact. The presence of elevated testosterone levels in addition to genetics could be the real risk factors for PCOS.

13.2.2.2.3 Monitoring FTM HT

Clinical monitoring should include regular examinations for the risk factors shown in Table 13.6. The FTM transsexual should be examined 3 months after any dosage increase or change and at least annually thereafter. Testosterone levels should be included in normal blood testing.

13.2.2.3 Mastectomy

FTM transsexuals typically start out by binding their breasts to look more masculine using tight fitting undergarments. Many FTM transsexuals eventually get a mastectomy or "top surgery" because of the discomfort of continuous binding and the need to be authentic. WPATH guidelines allow mastectomy to be conducted as early as the start of FTM HT.

13.2.2.4 Masculinization Surgery

Just as MTF get feminization surgery, so some FTM transsexuals get surgery to look more male. Many FTM transsexuals can avoid such surgery by growing beards to cover feminine features of the chin and cheeks.

13.2.2.5 Real-Life Experience

Before any FTM transsexual GPS is conducted, a yearlong RLE period is required by many surgeons to ensure that a FTM transsexual can live and work in a masculine gender behavior category. In most Western cultures, females can cross-dress without being rejected, so FTM transsexuals may already have adopting masculine clothing and eliminated feminine stimuli such as makeup and skirts before RLE. Because of HT, they may also already have facial hair. This eases the transition to RLE.

13.2.2.6 Transsexual GPS

Many FTM transsexuals have hysterectomies and salpingo-oophorectomies (removal of the Fallopian tubes and ovaries), but only 40% have transsexual GPS. There is a large variation of the procedure, depending on the needs of the FTM patient. In transsexual GPS, the urethra can be rerouted to empty through the clitoris that has been enlarged during HT. Various penile prostheses can be inserted to enlarge and lengthen the penis. A scrotum can also be created from the *labia majora* and prosthetic testicles can be implanted. Since erectile tissue and associated neural connections are not available for transsexual GPS, the genital change is often not as satisfactory as with MTF. Erectile prostheses are available but are not always satisfactory, and further research is needed to perfect them.

13.2.2.7 Voice Therapy

Although FTM HT lowers the fundamental frequency of the voice, FTM may seek voice therapy to eliminate feminine inflection and phraseology.

13.3 TRANSITION MORTALITY RISKS

Most of the mortality risks of transition seem to originate with the now passé use of ethinyl estradiol in MTF transsexuals, but studies have found increases in mortality from causes unrelated to transition. This suggests that although transsexual transition improves the well-being of FTM transsexuals, FTM transsexuals need continuous care for psychological and adjustment issues. In a study of FTM transsexuals in the Netherlands, Gooren (2008) found that mortality for both MTF and FTM was no different than for control subjects. However, there was a 6% to 8% increase in mortality for MTF transsexuals who took ethinyl estradiol, mostly due to venous thrombosis. Ethinyl estradiol has ceased to be prescribed for MTF HT in the Netherlands and most other countries.

Asscheman et al. (2011) found that mortality in MTF transsexuals was 51% higher than the general population, but death was from non-transition-related causes, primarily suicide, drug abuse, and HIV/AIDS. Use of ethinyl estradiol increased mortality from cardiovascular death threefold. Mortality for FTM was not increased. In Sweden, Dhejne et al. (2011) found a 4.5% increase in mortality for both MTF and FTM transsexuals, but the causes were unrelated to transition treatments. The major reason was from suicide. In Belgium, Wierckx et al. (2013) similarly found an increase in transsexual mortality over controls, and again, the main cause of the increase was suicide.

13.4 SEXUAL ORIENTATION OUTCOMES

Both MTF and FTM transition processes change the sexual orientation of some transsexuals. For MTF transsexuals, this change is noticed after transition is completed with transsexual GPS. For FTM transsexuals, the change seems to occur during HT and before transsexual GPS. Transsexuals and transgender people are a mixture of heterosexual, homosexual, and bisexual before transition (Bullough & Bullough, 1997). Bullough and Bullough (1997) reported that the MTF transgender population consisted of 67% attracted to females (heterosexual), 10.6% attracted to both sexes (bisexual), and 2.4% homosexual. The proportions in this mixture change after transsexual transition.

There have been two research studies reported that indicate that some MTF transsexuals change their sexual orientation from attraction to females to attraction to males after completing transition. The first study by Daskalos (1998) indicated that 6 of 20 MTF transsexuals reported changing sexual orientation and behavior. Lawrence (2005) conducted a larger study with 232 MTF transsexuals that found a shift from orientation to females to orientation to males of about 23%. Reports of the transsexuals indicated that preoperative sexual orientation was 54% to females, 9% to males, and 41% bisexual or asexual. Postoperative sexual orientation was 25% to females, 34% to males, and 37% bisexual or asexual. The Lawrence study indicated that 32% of the MTF transsexuals had not had a sexual partner within the past year. Bisexual MTF transsexuals had higher numbers of partners. In addition to the result indicating a shift in sexual orientation toward females, the study result of 25% remaining attracted to females supports the observation that some female significant others are able to adapt to their partner undergoing transition with sexual fluidity (Aramuru, 2013). This allows more heterosexual married couples to remain together after transition of the MTF transsexual.

The shift in sexual orientation among FTM transsexuals appears to begin during HT. Meier, Pardo, Labuski, and Babcock (2013) found in a study of 605 FTM transsexuals that 40% reported they had shifted their sexual orientation toward females during HT and continued after transition was completed. More than 50% reported that they were bisexual after transition.

13.5 TRANSITION AND TRANSSEXUAL GPS REGRET

Most MTF transsexuals report satisfaction after completing transition with transsexual GPS despite social adaptation problems and occasional postoperative complications (Lawrence, 2006). Transsexual transition is established as an effective treatment to improve the well-being of transsexuals (Kuiper & Cohen-Kettenis, 1988). Several large-scale studies have shown no adult MTF regret (Krege, Bex, Lummen, & Rubben, 2001; Lawrence, 2003; Lobato et al., 2006; Weyers et al., 2009). Others show a very low incidence of regret (3.8%; Landen, Walinder, Hambert, & Lundstrom, 1998). Transition during adolescence appears to increase satisfaction (Cohen-Kettenis & Goozen, 1997). Those MTF transsexuals who do regret transsexual GPS report family rejection or death of both parents (Lindemalm, Korlin, & Uddenberg, 1987) as the primary reasons. MTF transsexuals report satisfaction with hormone therapy (Gómez-Gil et al., 2012), although side effects have been reported.

FTM transsexuals also report satisfaction with completion of transition with transsexual GPS (Wierckx et al., 2011). FTM transsexuals also report satisfaction with hormone therapy (Constantino, Cerpolini, Morselli, Venturoli, & Merriggiola, 2013).

Transsexual transition is not a panacea, and the transsexual still faces significant social problems. Sometimes professional medical or mental health assistance is necessary. Overall, although transsexuals report satisfaction with completion of transition and transsexual GPS, they still have some quality of life (Kuhn et al., 2009) and sexual functioning difficulties (Lawrence, 2006).

13.6 SUMMARY

Transsexual transition appears to be a valuable treatment for transsexuals and transgender people who want to change their bodies to fit the associated sex of their congruent gender behavior category. Because there have been no comprehensive longitudinal studies of the effects of transition on transsexuals, many procedures are adjusted based on the judgment of mental health professionals, medical professionals, and the individual transsexual. Some of the procedures are ad hoc and vary with individual patients, such as the selection of drugs and dosages in HT. The primary role of mental health professionals in this process is to provide patient management and counseling and to be sure that the treatments are carried out in accordance with WPATH guidelines. Because transition involves swings of emotion due to new hormones and difficulties of social acceptance, counseling is often needed. There are some potential medical risks for both MTF and FTM transsexuals for which they should receive monitoring by medical professionals. To be safe, transsexual transition should not be a do-it-yourself proposition. Transsexual transition is the only known process that seems to change the sexual orientation of its participants. Few transsexuals express verbal regrets, but such regrets appear to be due to lack of acceptance by families and cultures.

REFERENCES

American College of Obstetrics and Gynecology. (2011, December). *Health care for transgender individuals* (no. 512). Retrieved March 27, 2014, from http://www.acog.org/~/media/Committee%20Opinions/Committee%20 on%20Health%20Care%20for%20Underserved%20Women/co512.pdf?d mc=1&ts=20140327T1953094088.

Aramuru, A. (2013). Relational and sexual fluidity in females partnered with male-to-female transsexual persons. *Journal of Psychiatric and Mental Health Nursing, 20,* 142–149.

Asscheman, H., Giltay, E., Megens, J., Ronde, W., Trotsenburg, M., & Gooren, L. (2011). Long-term follow-up study of mortality in transsexuals receiving treatment with cross-sex hormones. *European Journal of Endocrinology, 164*, 635–642.

Asscheman, H., Gooren, L. J., Assies, J., Smits, J. P., de Slegte, R. (1988). Prolactin levels and pituitary enlargement in hormone-treated male-to-female transsexuals. *Clin Endocrinal (OXF), 28*(6), 583–588.

Asscheman, H., Gooren, L., & Eklund, P. (1989). Mortality and morbidity in transsexual patients with cross-gender hormone treatment. *Metabolism, 38*, 869–873.

Asscheman, H., T'Sjoen, G., Lemaire, A., Mas, M., Merriggiola, M. C., Mueller, A., . . . Gooren, L. J. (2013). Venous thrombo-embolism as a complication of cross-sex hormone treatment of male-to-female transsexual subjects: A review [published online ahead of print August 14]. *Andrologia.*

Baba, T., Endo, T., Honnma, H., Kitajima, Y., Hayashi, T., Ikeda, H., . . . Saito, T. (2007). Association between polycystic ovary syndrome and female-male transsexuality. *Human Reproduction, 22*, 1011–1016.

Baron, S., Sowers, J., & Feinberg, M. (1983). Prolactinoma in a man following industrial exposure to estrogens. *Western Journal of Medicine, 138*, 720–722.

Bilefsky, D. (2012, July 23). *Serbia becomes a hub for sex-change surgery.* New York Times.

Buhrich, N. (1978). Motivation for cross-dressing in heterosexual transvestism. *Acta Psychiatrica Scandinavica, 57*, 145–152.

Bullough, B., & Bullough, V. (1997). Are transvestites necessarily heterosexual? *Archives of Sexual Behavior, 26*, 1–12.

Burnett, J. (2011a, September). *Harm reduction model for treatment of M2F TS below the poverty level—four year follow-up.* Presented at the WPATH Symposium 2011, Atlanta, GA.

Burnett, J. (2011b). *Cross gender hormone treatment for GID.* Presented at the Southern Comfort Conference.

Canadian Professional Association for Transgender Health. (2014). E-course in transgender endocrine therapy. CPATH & AstraZeneca Canada, Inc. Retrieved February 13, 2014, from http://www.isaixlearning.com/az /cours3/index_page.html.

Close, C. (2012). *Affirming gender, affirming lives: A report of the 2011 transition survey.* Santa Rosa, CA: Gender Advocacy Training and Education. Retrieved February 13, 2014, from http://transstudent.org/Affirming _Gender.pdf.

Cohen-Kettenis, P., & Goozen, S. (1997). Sex reassignment of adolescent transsexuals: A follow-up study. *Journal of the American Academy of Child and Adolescent Psychiatry, 26*, 263–271.

Constantino, A., Cerpolini, S., Morselli, P., Venturoli, S., & Merriggiola, M. (2013). A prospective study on sexual function and mood in female-to-male transsexuals during testosterone administration and after reassignment surgery. *Journal of Sex Marital Therapy, 39,* 321–325.

Daskalos, CT. (1998). Changes in the sexual orientation of six heterosexual male-to-female transsexuals. *Archives of Sexual Behavior, 27*(6), 605–615.

Davidson, A., Franicevich, J., Freeman, M., Lin, R., Martinez, L., Monihan, M., . . . Zevin, B. (2013). Protocols for hormonal reassignment of gender. Tom Waddell Health Center Transgender Team. Retrieved March 28, 2014, from http://www.sfdph.org/dph/comupg/oservices/medSvs /hlthCtrs/TransGendprotocols122006.pdf.

Dhejne, C., Lichtenstein, P., Boman, M., Johansson, V., Langstrom, N., & Landen, M. (2011). Long-term follow-up of transsexual persons undergoing sex reassignment surgery; cohort study in Sweden. *PLos ONE, 6,* e16885.

Fink, G. (1988). Oestrogen and progesterone interactions in the control of gonadotropin and prolactin secretion. *Journal of Steroid Biochemistry, 30,* 169–178.

Futterweit, W. (1998). Endocrine therapy of transsexuals: Potential complications of long-term treatment. *Archives of Sexual Behavior, 27,* 209–226.

Futterweit, W. (1999). Polycystic ovary syndrome: Clinical perspectives and management. *Obstetrics and Gynecology Survey, 54,* 403–413.

Futterweit, W., & Deligdisch, L. (1986). Histopathological effects of exogenously administered testosterone in 19 female to male transsexuals. *Journal of Clinical Endocrinology and Metabolism, 62,* 16–21.

Garcia-Malpartida, K., Martin-Gorgojo, A., Rocha, M., Gomez-Balaguer, M., & Hernandez-Mijares, A. (2010). Prolactinoma induced by estrogen and cyproterone acetate in a male-to-female transsexual. *Endocrinologia y Nutrción, 94,* e13–e15.

Gómez-Gil, E., Zubiaurre-Elorza, L., Esteva, I., Guillamon, A., Godás, T., Cruz Almaraz, M., . . . Salamero, M. (2012). Hormone-treated transsexuals report less social distress, anxiety and depression. *Psychoneuroendo, 37,* 662–670.

Gooren, L., Assies, J., Asscheman, H., de Slegte, R., & van Kessel, H. (1988). Estrogen-induced prolactinoma in a man. *Journal of Clinical Endocrinology and Metabolism, 66,* 444–446.

Gooren, L., Giltay, E., & Bunck, M. (2007). Long-term treatment of transsexuals with cross-sex hormones: Extensive personal experience. *Journal of Clinical Endocrinology and Metabolism, 93,* 19–25.

Gooren, L., Giltay, E. J., Bunck, M. C. (2008). Long-term treatment of transsexuals with cross-sex hormones. *Journal of Clinical Endocrinology & Metabolism, 93*(1), 19–25. DOI: 10.1210/jc.2007-1809.

Hembree, W. C., Cohen-Kettenis, P., Delemarre-van de Waal, H. A., Gooren, L. J., Meyer, W. J., III, Spack, N. P., . . . Montori, M. (2009). Endocrine treatment of transsexual persons: An Endocrine Society clinical practice guideline. *Journal of Clinical Endocrinology and Metabolism, 94,* 3132–3154.

Kovacs, K., Stefaneanu, L., Ezzat, S., & Smyth, H. (1994). Prolactin-producing pituitary adenoma in a male-to-female transsexual patient with protracted estrogen administration: A morphologic study. *Archives of Pathological Laboratory Medicine, 118*, 562–565.

Krege, S., Bex, A., Lummen, G., & Rubben, H. (2001). Male-female transsexualism: A technique, results and long-term follow-up in 66 patients. *BJU International, 88*, 396–402.

Kuhn, A., Bodmer, C., Stadimayr, W., Kuhn, P., Mueller, M., & Birkhauser, M. (2009). Quality of life 15 years after sex reassignment surgery for transsexualism. *Fertility and Sterility, 92*, 1685–1689.

Kuiper, B., & Cohen-Kettenis, P. (1988). Sex reassignment surgery: A study of 141 transsexuals. *Archives of Sexual Behavior, 17*, 439–457.

Landen, M., Walinder, J., Hambert, G., & Lundstrom, B. (1998). Factors predictive of regret in sex reassignment. *Acta Psychiatrica Scandinavica, 97*, 284–289.

Lawrence, A. (2003). Factors associated with satisfaction or regret following male-to-female sex reassignment surgery. *Archives of Sex Behavior, 32*, 299–315.

Lawrence, A. (2006). Patient-reported complications and functional outcomes of male-to-female sex reassignment surgery. *Archives of Sexual Behavior, 35*, 717–727.

Lawrence, A. (2005). Sexuality before and after male-to-female sex reassignment surgery. *Archives of Sexual Behavior, 34*, 147–166.

Lindemalm, G., Korlin, D., & Uddenberg, N. (1987). Prognostic factors vs. outcome in male-to-female transsexualism. A follow up study of 14 cases. *Acta Psychiatrica Scandinavica, 75*, 268–274.

Lobato, M. I., Koff, W. J., Manenti, C., da Fonseca Seger, D., Salvador, J., da Graça Borges Fortes, M., . . . Henriques, A. A. (2006). Follow-up of sex reassignment surgery in transsexuals: A Brazilian cohort. *Archives of Sexual Behavior, 35*, 711–715.

Lundberg, P., Sjovall, A., & Walinder, N. (1975). Sella turcica in male-to-female transsexuals. *Archives of Sexual Behavior, 4*, 657–662.

Meier, S., Pardo, S., Labuski, C., & Babcock, J. (2013). Measures of clinical health among female-to-male transgender persons as a function of sexual orientation. *Archives of Sexual Behavior, 42*, 463–474.

Mueller, A., Gooren, L., Nato-Schotz, S., Cupisti, S., Beckman, M., & Dittrich, R. (2008). Prevalence of polycystic ovary syndrome and hyperandrogenemia in female-to-male transsexuals. *Journal of Clinical Endocrinology and Metabolism, 93*, 1408–1411.

Olson, J. (2012, October 10). Treating transgender youth: Basics of cross-sex hormones. Strengthening Youth Prevention Paradigms at Children's Hospital Los Angeles. Retrieved February 13, 2014, from http://lachildrenshospital. net/webinar/SYPP_webinar_Olson_10_10_12/lib/playback.html.

Pache, T., & Fauser, B. (1993). Polycystic ovaries in female-to-male transsexuals. *Clinical Endocrinology (Oxf)*, *39*, 702–703.

Royal College of Psychiatrists. (1988). *Gender identity disorders in children and adolescents: Guidance for management* (Council Report CR63). London: Royal College of Psychatrists.

Schroeter, C., Groenewegen, J., Reinekie, T., & Neumann, H. (2003, September). Ninety percent permanent hair reduction in transsexual patients. *Annals of Plastic Surgery*, *51*, 243–248.

Serri, O., Noiseux, D., Robert, F., & Hardy, J. (1996). Lactotroph hyperplasia in an estrogen treated male-to-female transsexual patient. *Journal of Clinical Endocrinology and Metabolism*, *81*, 3177–3179.

Shipherd, J., Green, K., & Abramovitz, B. (2010). Transgender clients: Identifying and minimizing barriers to mental health treatment. *Journal of Gay & Lesbian Mental Health*, *14*, 94–108.

Tchaikovski, S. N., & Rosing, J. (2010). Mechanisms of estrogen-induced venous thromboembolism. *Thrombosis Research*, *126*, 5–11.

University of California at San Francisco Center of Excellence for Transgender Health. (2014). *Hormone administration*. UCSF Center of Excellence for Transgender Health. Retrieved February 14, 2014, from http://transhealth.ucsf.edu/trans?page=protocol-hormones.

U.S. Food and Drug Administration. (2011, June). *FDA update on the safety of silicone gel-filled breast implants*. FDA Center for Devices and Radiological Health. Retrieved February 13, 2014, from http://www.fda.gov/downloads/medicaldevices/productsandmedicalprocedures/implantsandprosthetics/breastimplants/UCM260090.pdf.

Van Caenegem, E., Taes, Y., Wierckx, K., Vandewalle, S., Toye, K., Kaufman, J.-M., & T'Sjoen, G. (2013, January 28). Low bone mass is prevalent in male-to-female transsexual persons before the start of cross-sex hormonal therapy and gonadectomy. *Bone*, *54*, 92–97.

Vroonen, L., Daly, A., & Beckers, A. (2013). Management of prolactinoma. *Revue Medecine Suisse*, *9*, 1522–1526.

Weyers, S., Elaut, E., De Sutter, P., Gerris, J., T'Sjoen, G., Heylens, G., . . . Verstraelen, H. (2009). Long-term assessment of the physical, mental, and sexual health among transsexual women. *Journal of Sexual Medicine*, *6*, 752–760.

Wibowo, E., Schellhammer, P., & Wassersug, R. (2011). Role of estrogen in normal male function: Clinical implications for patients with prostate cancer on androgen deprivation therapy. *Journal of Urology*, *185*, 17–23.

Wierckx, K., Anseeuw, E., Geerts, E., Elaut, E., Heylens, G., Motmans, J., Decuypere, G., & T'Sjoen, G. (2013). Cross-sex hormone therapy related adverse events: data from a large gender identity unit. *Endocrine Abstracts*, *32*, 969. DOI:10.1530/endoabs.32.P969

Wierckx, K., Elaut, E., Van Hoorde, B., Heylens, G., De Cuypere, G., Monstrey, S., . . . T'Sjoen, G. (2014). Sexual desire in trans persons: Associations with sex reassignment treatment. *Journal of Sexual Medicine, 11,* 107–118.

Wierckx, K., Mueller, S., Weyers, S., Van Caenegem, E., Roef, G., Heylens, G., & T'Sjoen, G. (2012). Long-term evaluation of cross-sex hormone treatment in transsexual persons. *Journal of Sexual Medicine, 9,* 2641–2651.

Wierckx, K., Van Caenegem, E., Elaut, E., Dedecker, D., Van de Peer, F., Toye, K., . . . T'Sjoen, G. (2011). Quality of life and sexual health after sex reassignment surgery in transsexual men. *Journal of Sexual Medicine, 8,* 3379–3388.

World Professional Association for Transgender Health (WPATH). (2013). *Standards of care.* Version 7. Retrieved September 2013 from http://www.wpath.org/publications_standards.cfm.

Xu, R., Wu, X., Di, A., Xu, J., Pang, C., & Pang, S. (2000). Pituitary prolactin-secreting tumor formulation: Recent developments. *Biological Signals and Receptors, 9,* 1–20.

Zelazniewicz, A., & Pawlowski, B. (2011). Female breast size attractiveness for men as a function of sociosexual orientation (restricted vs. unrestricted). *Archives of Sexual Behavior, 40,* 1129–1135.

Conclusion

14.0 THE REST OF WILLIAM'S STORY

Like other parents, John and Jane Doe both contributed DNA to make William. Either John or Jane may have passed on a genetic pattern for transsexualism and transgenderism (TSTG) from their ancestors, or at conception a de novo mutation might have occurred that neither parent possessed. Like other parents, John and Jane pass on other non-DNA chemicals to their offspring that could have altered the expression of William's DNA. Passage of such chemicals, known as imprinting, has been detected in the ratio of aunts to uncles on the maternal side for transsexuals.

Although mothers like Jane are now more aware of the deleterious effects that drugs and chemicals can have on the developing fetus, not so many years ago, these effects were unknown. In Jane's case, she found out late in her pregnancy so William might have been exposed to her antiseizure medication while in her womb. There are other drugs and chemicals in the environment that also cause epigenetic effects, but none of these are established as being involved in TSTG. Chemical spills can penetrate into the water and food supply from rivers and streams, and these chemicals can persist for weeks and months.

We know that maternal stress can cause genetic mutations and changes in DNA expression, so when Jane was stressed by getting the flu during her pregnancy, it might have contributed to the epigenetic effects. It is true that the flu shot you take today will only protect you from last year's flu because it takes several months for this year's virus to be characterized and used to make a vaccine. When both John and Jane at one point lost their jobs, this increased the maternal stress on Jane, which may also have influenced expression of William's DNA.

Children begin to realize that they are transsexual or transgender at about age 4, leaving little time for factors other than genetics and epigenetics to be causal factors in TSTG. William's choice of playthings was perfectly normal, but his tendancy to use with his left hand is consistent with transsexuals who are less right-handed.

Transsexual and transgender children typically get their first experience with cross-dressing in the home, and William was no exception. Although they know the rules of each gender behavior category starting at about age 2, children are drawn to the gender behavior category that is congruent with their gender predisposition. William was attracted to feminine clothing and makeup and gradually started playing exclusively with his mother's and not his father's things. William, like other children, knew the pink-blue gender behavior category rule by age 2 or 3, yet asking for a pink birthday party hat was natural to him.

When William told his parents that he was a girl, not a boy, and expressed his rage that he could not be with the girls in the kindergarten class, he was being honest about his TSTG, for perhaps the last time in childhood. He got a lecture about how he was supposed to behave in his assigned masculine gender behavior category and what was expected in the future. However, in a few months, he had already adopted a strategy of secrecy to avoid parental rejection and teacher punishment. He did his cross-dressing in secret so that he could not be discovered.

William got the message that it was not safe for him to behave like a girl, even though he was drawn to behave that way. He decided that he would stop talking about being a girl to his parents and others and just be a girl in private. He could sneak into his mother's room and borrow her clothing. He now knew how to take off makeup with tissue and makeup remover. He could now put on makeup and quickly take it off when he was in the locked bathroom. He would play along in school and at church. He would keep his secret from everyone. Like many transsexual and transgender children and adults, he could only express behavior from his congruent gender behavior category in private.

High school is a particularly trying time for transsexual and transgender children. In addition to going through puberty, they must master a gender behavior category that is not congruent with their gender predisposition or adopt a strategy of secrecy. William could see how boys who looked feminine or behaved in a feminine manner were bullied and attacked. As many male-to-female children do, William displayed masculine behavior and participated in "manly sports" to divert attention from his secret TSTG activities.

The result of such secrecy is inauthenticity, depression, self-isolation, illness, and sometimes suicide.

William began to hang out with the girls because he felt more comfortable with them. He would observe their feminine presentation and behavior carefully because it was what he wanted to perform. But by observing their behavior carefully, he was exposing himself to sexual arousal learning to stimuli associated with the feminine gender behavior category. Because his male body was prone to become aroused spontaneously, he became conditioned to get aroused by these feminine stimuli. He was not safe from getting aroused, even in his sleep when the wet dreams would come.

William finished school, got a job, became independent, and moved into an apartment. The apartment was small, but it gave him absolute privacy. William, like other transsexual and transgender people, started out with individual pieces of clothing and makeup but rapidly moved to complete cross-dressing. William could also dress as Billie on business trips. This is the perfect type of situation to practice feminine dress and behavior for many transsexual and transgender people, but eventually the need to be with other transsexual and transgender people to "compare notes" becomes overwhelming. It is at this point that many begin first to join online discussions, then to go to safe support group meetings, and then to safe bars and other public places. William would go on occasional dates so that he could join discussions at work about his "love life." This was another means of diverting attention from his secretive "hobby" and is common among transsexual and transgender people.

William met Linda at work and fell in love. Like so many transgender people, William believed that marriage would "cure" him of his TSTG behavior. This is known as "marriage flight." Homosexuality appears to be independent from TSTG so marrying a natal female is common for male-to-female (MTF) transsexuals and transgender people. There is also, for some, "military flight" in which transsexual and transgender people believe that the burden of their secrecy will be lifted by becoming involved in such a risky occupation. Transsexual and transgender people join the military with twice the frequency as other people.

After the wedding, William faced a common problem of transgender people, that of "purging" his opposite sex clothes and makeup. Transgender people purge periodically in the hope that their TSTG will go away or at least the probability of discovery will be temporarily eliminated. But soon they typically acquire another collection of cross-gender clothing. This cycle is repeated, especially at points of life change, such as getting married to Linda.

Although TSTG ultimately does seem to be motivated by the pursuit of sexual arousal and satisfaction, transsexual and transgender people do initially get aroused by cross-dressing. Sexual arousal lessens with repeated cross-dressing. As it did for William, this resulted in reduced sexual arousal in bed with Linda.

Big changes in TSTG behavior are sometimes triggered by life events. (Such life events also change the behavior of nontranssexual and nontransgender people as well.) Life events trigger one of four kinds of "existential crisis," which is frequently resolved by changes in behavior. William was seriously injured in an automobile accident, which triggered two existential crises. William realized that life was too short to keep his cross-dressing a secret (mortality). He felt guilty that he was deceiving his wife (isolation). He sat down with Linda and told her about Billie. Linda, like most "significant others" (SOs) was confused and scared. Her feelings included sympathy for her spouse, anger at his deceptions, and doubt about her own sexuality, and these feelings were difficult to handle. Mental health professionals who have experience with TSTG can provide counseling. Linda also took advantage of other sources of help, including literature and SO support groups.

Linda went through more periods of confusion and panic, wondering whether William would become a transsexual. This is common for SOs. William could not totally comfort her because he did not know what he would do in the future. William and Linda stayed together because they still loved each other and their child. But they were uncertain about the future. William could now go to the local support group instead of those out of town and be with his transgender friends, this time with his wife's knowledge and sometimes participation. If William decides to transition as a transsexual, it is now possible William and Linda may stay together. Early transition rules required transsexuals to divorce, but those rules have now been relaxed.

Although this is a typical life history of a transgender person, several variations are not uncommon:

- William's parents could have been more accepting and allowed him to have a "social transition" as a child with guidance from a mental health professional. The social transition concept is relatively new. A social transition allows a transsexual or transgender person to follow a congruent gender behavior category and cross-dress to determine whether a feminine gender was right for him. Social transitions are usually for those TSTG children who believe that they may be transsexuals.
- In recent years, the child's social transition could have been accompanied by the administration of "blocker hormones" to delay puberty and give William more time to decide about Billie.
- If puberty was delayed, William could have started transsexual transition to feminize his body as early as age 16.
- William could have spontaneously decided at any time in his life that he was a transsexual and started transition, with either the approval and assistance of a mental health professional or following the dangerous "do-it-yourself" route.

- William could have gone into the military, become a fireman, or become a missionary to occupy himself with a socially acceptable vocation that required intense concentration and would compete with his transgender behavior.
- William might not have had the automobile accident, and he would not come out to Linda.

14.1 THE BIOPSYCHOLOGY OF TSTG

So, briefly, what do we know about TSTG from a biopsychology perspective?

We know that transsexuals and transgender people are more common in the population than was previously thought. Early estimates of population frequency were based on counting those who attend TSTG clinics. More recently, mathematical estimation techniques and population surveys indicate that the frequency is several orders of magnitude higher.

We know that there are substantial human and cultural costs for rejecting transsexual and transgender people. The human costs often involve secrecy that causes loss of authenticity, self-enforced isolation, loss of self-esteem, depression, and sometimes suicide. They also include micro-aggressions, bullying, and physical violence. It is hoped that scientific knowledge of TSTG will reduce these costs by providing a factual basis for public policy and interpersonal understanding.

TSTG is a phenomenon in which the gender behavior or verbal declaration of gender identity of individuals is incongruent with their assigned natal gender behavior category and congruent with some other gender behavior category. Gender behavior category is typically determined by natal sex, but some cultures also use gender identity as well.

We know that TSTG is probably a biological phenomenon because of the historical and geographic spread of gender diversity and cultural accommodation. Information from genetics and epigenetics, as well as the appearance of TSTG in early childhood and other evidence, confirms that it is biological in nature.

Looking at the spread of gender diversity across cultures, we understand that cultures form gender behavior categories, sometimes more than two and up to five. Culture typically assigns people to one of these categories. The assigned category may not be congruent with a person's biological gender predisposition. The result is TSTG. Some cultures allow movement between gender behavior categories, such as those with a two-spirit tradition.

Evidence from biopsychology indicates that the two causal factors for TSTG appear to be genetics and epigenetics, perhaps working together. We know genetics is involved because of twin and family studies and genetic markers on the DNA molecule for TSTG. We believe epigenetics may be

involved because TSTG is implicated as being correlated with such phenomena as prenatal exposure to drugs. Prenatal exposure to toxic chemicals and
maternal stress are also potential epigenetic mechanisms for TSTG. Genetic
and epigenetic factors may work together to produce a gender predisposition
that may be incongruent with cultural expectations of a person's appropriate
gender behavior category. We know that the prenatal testosterone theory of
TSTG causation is not supported by the evidence. Several phenomena are
known to involve both genetics and epigenetics, and TSTG is correlated with
some of them. In particular, transsexuals and transgender people tend to be
less right-handed. Genetic and epigenetic evidence as well as absence of evidence for other causal factors forms the basis for the two-factor theory of
TSTG causation.

We know that both understanding of gender behavior categories and realization of TSTG occur at early childhood ages. Most children have grasped
the fundamentals of the gender system in which they live by age 2 or 3. Realization of TSTG starts at about age 4 or 5. Some children may not be able to
articulate their realization, but they know something is different about themselves at an early age. Once they realize that TSTG behavior results in parental and cultural rejection, many children adopt a strategy of secrecy that may
extend into adulthood.

There is no evidence that improper child rearing or adverse parent-child
relationships are causal factors in TSTG. Transsexual and transgender children are subject to parental violence, however, which is probably a result of
parental rejection of TSTG behavior. We understand that parents now have
additional options for dealing with transsexual and transgender children.
The first is to conduct a social transition in childhood and live in their congruent gender behavior category. The second is to combine social transition
with delaying puberty using blocker hormones. This latter option allows for
a smooth social transition and gives all concerned more time to determine
whether and when transsexual transition might begin.

We understand that sexual arousal is learned and that it can be extinguished by repeated exposure according to the rules of classical, or Pavlovian, conditioning. Transsexuals and transgender people do initially become
aroused by cross-dressing and cross-presentation, but this arousal decreases
rapidly with exposure. TSTG behavior persists despite this decline in arousal,
which indicates that TSTG is not a sexual fetish. Reports indicate that transgender people cross-dress for relaxation, not sexual arousal.

Science shows that there are anatomical and neurophysiological markers for TSTG, providing further evidence that TSTG is biological in nature.
Markers include less right-handedness, finger length ratio, and female-to-
male (FTM) biometrics. Neuroanatomical and neurophysiological differences have also been identified for TSTG.

We also know that situations creating existential crises may result in transsexual and transgender people increasing their cross-dressing frequency, induce them to come more out of the closet, or impel them to go into transsexual transition. Existential crises are triggered by realization of mortality or the intrinsic meaninglessness of life. Other existential crises are triggered by the realization of the crushing responsibility that one is responsible to fix everything wrong in the world or feelings of isolation from other people. Examples of such triggers are loss of a loved one, particularly a spouse; resolution of a medical crisis; the end of a war; or the end of a long-term endeavor. We understand that existential crises frequently change behavior, whether TSTG or other behaviors.

TSTG is not a conscious lifestyle choice. Subconscious mechanisms make choices for us before there is any conscious awareness of them. Decisions regarding TSTG are influenced by biological gender predisposition, fear of exposure, and decisions about existential crises and other things, all of which are represented somewhere in the subconscious.

Although spirituality is one of the most important experiences in human existence, we can find no evidence of an ethereal spirit that controls our brain and thus our behavior. Scientists and others have been looking for an interface between an ethereal spirit and human physiology since antiquity, but especially since Descartes' advocacy in the 1600s. Given the way ethereal spirits have been defined, such an interface would be self-contradictory because it would violate ethereality or corporeal rules. Someday we may find such an interface, but for now, if spirituality can be gendered as two-spirits report, we must conclude that gendered spirituality resides in subconscious mechanisms. This is not to reject spirituality but only to state the status of our science.

We know that mental health professionals have been and are on the front line of helping transsexuals and transgender people with their problems. Because they are schooled in the "medical model," they have tried to apply various pathological theories to explain transsexual and transgender behavior. The medical model requires such theories to determine appropriate treatment. Most of these theories involved intervening variables and phenomena that were not observable or measurable, and most were not scientific theories in that they could not be operationalized or make definitive predictions so that they could be tested. Given the rapid improvements in medical science and instrumentation and better understanding of physiological phenomena, it should now be possible to observe TSTG functionality in the brain. We can then begin to develop scientific theories of TSTG that can be tested and devise evidence-based treatments.

We know that some people follow the path of transsexual transition. Transsexual transition is effective, and most transsexuals report satisfaction.

Transsexuals and medical professionals should be aware of the specific medical risks and monitor their patients accordingly. Only about 25% to 40% of transsexuals actually receive TS genital plastic surgery (GPS). About 23% of MTF transsexuals change their sexual orientation after TS GPS. FTM transsexuals also change their sexual orientation but do so earlier than MTF, at the beginning of HT.

Improved understanding of TSTG can be obtained from scientific evidence. But understanding can be accelerated by establishing interpersonal relationships between transsexual and transgender people and the rest of the population. This requires that transsexuals and transgender people become more visible and, armed with the scientific facts, reach out to nontranssexual and nontransgender people.

Appendix A

Suggestions for Further Reading

ADVOCACY

National Center for Transgender Equality (NCTE). (2009). *Injustice at every turn.* Retrieved February 26, 2014, from http://transequality.org/PDFs /Executive_Summary.pdf.

National Center for Transgender Equality (NCTE). (2012). *A blueprint for equality: A federal agenda for transgender people.* Retrieved February 26, 2014, from http://transequality.org/Resources/NCTE_Blueprint_for_ Equality2012_FINAL.pdf.

AUTOBIOGRAPHY

Bevan, D. (2012). *The transsexual scientist.* Amazon Books.

Boylan, J. (2013). *She's not here: A life in two genders.* New York: Broadway Books.

Eugenides, J. (2002). *Middlesex.* New York: Picador.

Morris, J. (1974). *Conundrum.* New York: Signet.

CHILDREN

Brill, S. (2008). *The transgender child.* Cleis Press/Kindle.

Ehrensaft, D. (2011). *Gender born, gender made, raising healthy gender nonconforming children.* Kindle/Amazon Digital Services.

Ewert, M. (2008). *10,000 dresses*. New York City: Seven Stories Press.
Kildavis, C. (2002). *My princess boy*. New York: Aladdin.

CLINICAL PSYCHOLOGY

Lev, A. (2004). *Transgender emergence*. New York: Haworth Press.

CULTURES

Brown, L. (1997). *Two spirit people: American Indian lesbian woman and gay men*. New York: Routledge.
Costa, L., & Matzner, A. (2007). *Male bodies, women's souls: Personal narratives of Thailand's transgendered youth*. New York: Routledge.
Jacobs, S., Thomas, W., & Lang, S. *Two-spirit people*. Urbana: University of Illinois Press.
Nanda, S. (2000). *Gender diversity: Crosscultural variations*. Prospect Heights, IL: Waveland.
Roscoe, W. (1998). *Changing ones: Third and fourth genders in native North America*. New York: St. Martin's Griffin.
Williams, W. *The spirit and the flesh: Sexual diversity in American Indian Culture*. Boston: Beacon.

FAMILY

Boylan, J. (2013). *Stuck in the middle with you—a memoir of parenting in three genders*. New York: Broadway Books.

HISTORY

Stryker, S. (2008). *Transgender history*. Berkeley, CA: Perseus.
Verstaete, B., & Provencal, V. (2005). *Same-sex desire and love in Greco-Roman antiquity and in the Classical tradition of the West*. New York: Harrington Park Press.

PHILOSOPHY

Bornstein, K. (1995). *Gender outlaw: On men, women and the rest of us*. New York: Vintage.
Evatt, C. (2008). *The myth of free will*. Sausalito, CA: Café Essays.

Ryle, G., & Dennett, D. (2012). *The concept of mind.* Chicago: University of Chicago Press.

SCIENCE

Brill, S., & Pepper, R. (2008). *The transgender child: A handbook for families and professionals.* Berkeley, CA: Cleis Press.

Colapinto, J. (2002). *As nature made him: The boy who was raised as a girl.* New York: Perennial.

Devor, H. (1997). *FTM: Female-to-male transsexuals in society.* Bloomington: Indiana University Press.

Jaynes, J. (2000). *The origin of consciousness in the breakdown of the bicameral mind.* New York: Houghton.

Kelly, A. (2002). *The psychology of secrets.* New York: Plenum.

Migeon, B. (2007). *Females are mosaics: X-inactivation and sex differences in disease.* New York: Oxford University Press.

Roughgarden, J. (2004). *Evolutions rainbow: Diversity, gender and sexuality in nature and people.* Berkeley: University of California Press.

SELF-HELP

Denny, D. (1997). *Identity management in transsexualism.* Creative Design Services.

Prince, V. (1979). *How to be a woman though male.* Washington DC: Chevalier Publications.

Prince, V. (1976). *Understanding cross-dressing.* CA: Sandy Thomas Publications.

Rudd, P. (2011). *Crossdressing with dignity.* Katy, TX: PM Publishers.

SIGNIFICANT OTHERS

Erhardt, V. (2007). *Head over heels: Wives that stay with cross-dressers and transsexuals.* London: Haworth.

Rudd, P. (1999). *My husband wears my clothes.* Katy, TX: PM Publishers.

TEEN

Alden, J. (2013). *A season for April, Part 1: Summer Storms.* Kindle/Amazon Digital Services.

Amato, R. (2014). *I'm your daughter too.* Createspace Independent Publishing Platform.

Krieger, I. (2011). *Helping your transgender teen: A guide for parents.* Kindle/Amazon Digital Services.

Kuklin, S. (2014). *Beyond magenta: Transgender teens speak out.* Kindle/Amazon Digital Services.

Peters, J. (2002). *Luna: A novel.* New York: Megan Tingley Books.

WORKPLACE

Weiss, J. (2007). *Transgender workplace diversity.* Charleston, SC: Booksurge.

Appendix B

Organizations Serving Transsexuals and Transgender People

ADVOCACY

Gay and Lesbian Medical Association. Retrieved February 15, 2014, from http://www.glma.org/index.cfm?fuseaction=Page.viewPage&pageId=532.

Gender Education and Advocacy. Retrieved February 15, 2014, from http://www.ftmi.org.

National Center for Transgender Equality. Retrieved February 15, 2014, from http://transequality.org.

Organisation Intersex International Australia. Retrieved February 15, 2014, from http://oii.org.au.

Out and Equal. Retrieved February 15, 2014, from http://outandequal.org/town-calls.

EDUCATION

Association for Gender Research, Academia and Action. Retrieved February 15, 2014, from http://agreaa.org.

Gender Spectrum. Retrieved February 15, 2014, from https://www.genderspectrum.org.

International Federation for Gender Education. Retrieved February 15, 2014, from http://www.ifge.org.

Susan's Place. Retrieved February 15, 2014, from http://www.susans.org.

ELDERLY TRANSGENDER PEOPLE

FORGE. Retrieved February 15, 2014, from http://forge-forward.org.
Services & Advocacy for GLBT Elders (SAGE). Retrieved February 15, 2014, from http://www.sageusa.org.

FAMILY

Family Acceptance Project. San Francisco State University. Retrieved February 15, 2014, from http://familyproject.sfsu.edu.
Female to Male International. Retrieved February 15, 2014, from http://www.ftmi.org.
PFLAG. Retrieved February 15, 2014, from http://community.pflag.org/Page.aspx?pid=194&srcid=-2.
Trans Youth Family Allies. Retrieved February 15, 2014, from http://www.imatyfa.org.

HEALTH CARE

American Psychological Association. Retrieved February 15, 2014, from http://www.apa.org/pi/lgbt/programs/transgender/15.
American Psychiatric Association. Retrieved February 15, 2014, from http://www.psych.org.
Center of Excellence for Transgender Health, University of California San Francisco. Retrieved February 15, 2014, from http://transhealth.ucsf.edu.
Children's National Health System. Retrieved February 15, 2014, from http://www.childrensnational.org.
National Coalition for LGBT Health. Retrieved February 15, 2014, from http://lgbthealth.webolutionary.com/about.
SYPP Center at Children's Hospital, Los Angeles. Retrieved February 15, 2014, from http://www.chla.org/site/c.ipINKTOAJsG/b.6092439/k.1F71/Center_for_Strengthening_Youth_Prevention_Paradigms__SYPP__HIV_Prevention__AtRisk_Youth__Webinars.htm#.Uv--UHlXGkQ.
Tavistock Clinic, London, UK. Retrieved February 15, 2014, from http://www.tavistockandportman.nhs.uk.
World Professional Association for Transgender Health. Retrieved February 15, 2014, from http://www.wpath.org.

LEGAL

Lambda Legal. Retrieved February 15, 2014, from http://www.lambdalegal.org
Sylvia Rivera Law Project. Retrieved February 15, 2014, from http://srlp.org.

Transgender Law Center. Retrieved February 15, 2014, from http://
   transgenderlawcenter.org.

MEDIA

GLAAD. Retrieved February 15, 2014, from http://www.glaad.org.
Transmedia Media Watch, UK. Retrieved February 15, 2014, from http://
   www.transmediawatch.org.

MEETINGS

Colorado Gold Rush, Denver, CO. Retrieved February 15, 2014, from http://
   www.gicofcolo.org.
Esprit, Port Angeles, WA. Retrieved February 15, 2014, from http://www
   .espritconf.com.
First Event, Peabody, MA. Retrieved February 15, 2014, from http://firstevent
   .org.
Gender Odyssey, Seattle, WA. Retrieved February 15, 2014, from http://www
   .genderodyssey.org.
Keystone Conference, Harrisburg, PA. Retrieved February 15, 2014, from
   http://transcentralpa.org/keystone.htm.
Philadelphia Trans-Health Conference, Philadelphia, PA. Retrieved February
   15, 2014, from http://www.trans-health.org.
Southern Comfort Conference, Atlanta, GA. Retrieved February 15, 2014,
   from http://sccatl.org/content.
Sparkle, Manchester, UK. Retrieved February 15, 2014, from http://www
   .sparkle.org.uk.
Fantasia Fair, Provincetown, RI. Retrieved February 15, 2014, from http://
   www.fantasiafair.org.

SIGNIFICANT OTHERS, FAMILY, FRIENDS, AND ALLIES OF FTM

FTM Information Network. Retrieved February 15, 2014, from http://www
   .ftminfo.net/soffa.html.

SUPPORT GROUPS

Beaumont Society, UK. Retrieved February 15, 2014, from http://www
   .beaumontsociety.org.uk/Index.html.
Renaissance, Philadelphia. Retrieved February 15, 2014, from http://www
   .ren.org/rafil/gpc/gpc.html.

Tiffany Club of New England. Retrieved February 15, 2014, from http://tcnetg.wpengine.com.

Transgender Educational Association of greater Washington. Retrieved February 15, 2014, from http://www.tgea.net.

Tri Ess, US. Retrieved February 15, 2014, from http://www.tri-ess.org/index.html.

Seahorse Society of New South Wales. Retrieved March 31, 2014, from http://www.seahorsesoc.org/index.html.

Susan's Place Support Group Listing. Retrieved February 15, 2014, from http://www.susans.org/Local_Support_Groups_and_Organizations.

VOICE

Exceptional Voice. (Kathe Perez). 930 W 7th Avenue, Suite B, Denver, CO 80204-4444. Retrieved April 4, 2014, http://www.exceptionalvoice.com.

Index

adolescent and young adult, 153–159; family and cultural rejection, 156; gender task learning, 153–153; military and marriage flight, 158–159; outcomes, 157–158; secrecy and discontinuation, 157; sexual arousal learning, 154–156

androgen insensitivity syndrome (AIS), 78; definition, 78; mutations of androgen receptor gene involvement, 90–91, 96–97; refutation of PTTT, 115

androgen receptor gene, 78–79; definition, 78–79; effects of prenatal environment on, 110, 127; marker for androgen insensitivity syndrome (AIS), 91; marker for non-right handedness, 126; marker for TSTG, 78, 86–90

antiquity, 66–67; castrati, 66–67; castration, 69; Corded Ware culture, 66; eunuchs, 66–67; Queen Hatshepsut, 66; TSTG in, 66–67

Asian and Pacific cultures gender behavior categories, 71–74; Hawaiian *mahu*, 73; Indonesian *bugis*, 73–74; Indonesian *bugis* and spirituality, 178; Indonesian *waria*, 72–73; Indonesian *waria* and Barack Obama, 71–73; Philippines *bakla*, 73; Samoan *fa'afafine*, 73; South Asia *hirja*, 72; Thailand *kathoey*, 72

authenticity, 18–20; definition, 18; human cost of TSTG rejection, 15; need for TS transition, 210

autogynephilia, 191–194; core scale, 193; definition, 191–192; pathologization of TSTG, 191, 194; peer review criticism, 193–194; phalloplethysmograph experiment, 193; remains in DSM-V, 10, 201; sexual fetish, 191; variety of definitions, 192

Benjamin, Harry, 42

Biber, Stanley, 222

biological imperative, 10, 180–184, 186; illusion of conscious choice, 182–184; nervous system mechanisms, 184; subconscious mechanisms are out of control, xi–xii

biopsychology, 6; aids definition of terms across sciences, 7, 37; definition, 6; organization of scientific evidence, 6; provides power, xii; summary for TSTG, 241–244

About the Author

THOMAS E. BEVAN, PhD, is an experimental psychologist who conducts biopsychology research on transsexualism and transgenderism. He held the rank of professor and taught biopsychology at the Georgia Institute of Technology. He has developed biopsychology applications for the military including a telemedicine system for the U.S. Marine Corps to assist in the treatment of casualties of weapons of mass destruction and a biopsychology-based medical training system, for which he won a U.S. Army Innovation award. Bevan received a BA from Dartmouth College, majoring in experimental psychology, and a PhD from Princeton University in physiological psychology.